C000150322

Mark L Levy MBChB (Pretoria), FRCGP
General Practitioner (London) and GPIAG Editor
Kenton Bridge Medical Centre, Kenton, Harrow, UK

Linda Pearce MSc, RN, SCM, OHNc, NPdip
Respiratory Nurse Consultant
Department of Respiratory Medicine, West Suffolk
Hospital, Bury St Edmunds, Suffolk, UK

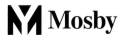

MOSBY
An imprint of Elsevier Limited

© 2004 Elsevier Limited. All rights reserved.

No part of this publication may be reproduced, stored in a retrieval
system, or transmitted in any form or by any means, electronic,
mechanical, photocopying, recording or otherwise, without either the
prior permission of the publishers or a licence permitting restricted
copying in the United Kingdom issued by the Copyright Licensing
Agency, 90 Tottenham Court Road, London W1T 4LP. Permissions
may be sought directly from Elsevier's Health Sciences Rights
Department in Philadelphia, USA: phone: (+1) 215 238 7869, fax: (+1)
215 238 2239, e-mail: healthpermissions@elsevier.com. You may also
complete your request on-line via the Elsevier homepage
(http://www.elsevier.com), by selecting 'Customer Support' and then
'Obtaining Permissions'.

First published 2004
    Reprinted 2004, 2005

ISBN 0 7234 3360 7

British Library Cataloguing in Publication Data
A catalogue record for this book is available from the British Library

Library of Congress Cataloguing in Publication Data
A catalogue record for this book is available from the Library of
Congress

Note
Medical knowledge is constantly changing. As new information
becomes available, changes in treatment, procedures, equipment and
the use of drugs become necessary. The editors, contributor and the
publishers have taken care to ensure that the information given in this
text is accurate and up to date. However, readers are strongly advised
to confirm that the information, especially with regard to drug usage,
complies with the latest legislation and standards of practice.

The authors would like to thank Professor Martyn Partridge of the
BTS/ Sign and Monica Fletcher of the NRTC for permission to
reproduce a significant number of figures and tables in this book.

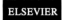

ELSEVIER your source for books,
journals and multimedia
in the health sciences

www.elsevierhealth.com

Working together to grow
libraries in developing countries
www.elsevier.com | www.bookaid.org | www.sabre.org

ELSEVIER   BOOKAID
International   Sabre Foundation

The
Publisher's
policy is to use
**paper manufactured
from sustainable forests**

Printed in China

Acknowledgements

I dedicate this book to my wife Celia. Her love, support and sense of humour sustain me.

Mark Levy

With grateful thanks to Phil, David, Phillip and Paul for their help, support and understanding.

Linda Pearce

Foreword

The late Professor Ann Wolcoock once said: "Asthma is like love, everybody knows what it is but nobody can define it". This excellent book, written by Mark L Levy and Linda Pearce, not only defines asthma in a simple straight forward way, it also provides much practical assistance to general practitioners and asthma nurses on how to diagnose, monitor and treat asthma. All relevant subjects are dealt with and very clearly explained. Many practical examples are given on improving compliance and self-management by patients. The book is very readable, complete and up to date. Especially helpful for the practitioner is the last chapter on frequently asked questions. I can advise everybody to read this book and to use it for daily care.

Professor Onno van Schayck
University of Maastricht
Department of General Practice

Contents

Abbreviations

BDP	beclomethasone dipropionate
BGAM	British Guidelines on Asthma Management
BHR	bronchial hyper-responsiveness
BTS	British Thoracic Society
BUD	budesonide
cAMP	cyclic 3',5'-adenosine monophosphate
CARAS	combined allergic rhinitis and asthma syndrome
cGMP	cyclic 3',5'-guanosine monophosphate
COPD	chronic obstructive pulmonary disease
COX	cyclo-oxygenase
DPI	dry powder inhaler
FEV_1	forced expiratory volume in the first second of expiration
FP	fluticasone propionate
FVC	forced vital capacity
GINA	Global Initiative on Asthma
GPIAG	General Practice Airways Group
IgE	immunoglobulin E
LABA	long-acting b_2-agonist
LTRA	leukotriene receptor antagonist
MF	mometasone furoate
NSAID	non-steroidal anti-inflammatory drug
PEF	peak expiratory flow
pMDI	pressurized metered dose inhaler
RCGP	Royal College of General Practitioners
sIgE	allergen-specific immunoglobulin E
SIGN	Scottish Intercollegiate Guidelines Network

Introduction

Asthma is one of the commonest chronic diseases worldwide, with evidence that the prevalence is increasing, particularly in the case of children. Up to 2% of health care costs in western countries are spent on asthma management. This cost will become an increasing burden for developing countries as atopy and asthma increase. The UK prevalence of asthma in males increased by 114% and in females by 165% between the 1980s and the 1990s,[1] and the cost of respiratory disease to the National Health Service is higher than in any other disease area, at an estimated £2.5 billion in the year 2000, with around two-fifths of these costs (£1 billion) being for in-patient care.[1]

Although deaths from asthma in the UK have declined over the past decade, over 1500 people still die due to the illness each year; this includes 25 children and 500 adults under 65 years.[2] Many of these deaths are considered by experts to be preventable.[3]

Health care utilization due to inadequate or poor asthma control comprises a major economic burden for Primary Care Organizations, who are extremely short of funds. Almost 4 million consultations and 74,000 hospital admissions for asthma each year in the UK account for an estimated annual cost of asthma to the NHS of over £850 million.[2]

Despite the development and acceptance of international guidelines, asthma remains under-diagnosed and, even when diagnosed, many people accept poorly controlled asthma and interference with daily activity and sleep disturbance as a normal part of their disease. This morbidity results in considerable absence from school and work, adding to the national economic burden.

The organization of structured care is important, and there is good evidence to suggest that trained health professionals could provide better outcomes for patients through improved management of this chronic disease.

This could be achieved by increasing the uptake of training in asthma management by health professionals. In the UK, this would require much more input and direction from Primary Care Organizations as well as the Government, which has been sadly lacking in the last 2 decades.

Proactive approaches to the use of preventative medications and effective management have the potential to reduce morbidity and mortality. Working in partnership with patients may greatly enhance asthma care, assisted by greater distribution and uptake of action plans aimed at empowering patients to take more control of their disease.

This book provides a practical, evidence-based approach to asthma management.

Definition and Epidemiology

Asthma is defined as "a chronic inflammatory disorder of the airways in susceptible individuals". Inflammatory symptoms are usually associated with widespread but variable airflow obstruction and an increase in airway response to a variety of stimuli.[4]

Asthma may be allergic or non-allergic. In general, epidemiological studies tend to define asthma in one of two ways, either the self-reporting or physician diagnosis of asthma-like symptoms (e.g. wheezing at rest or on exertion, dyspnoea at rest, chest tightness or cough) or bronchial hyper-responsiveness as defined by a positive result to a bronchial challenge test. Asthma may be subdivided further in terms of severity or response to specific triggers (e.g. dust, pollen, animal dander, tobacco smoke).

Asthma morbidity, its prevalence and incidence, is measured by outcomes such as patient symptoms and quality of life, severity, use of medication and utilization of health services.

Morbidity

Patient surveys and questionnaires over the past 10 years demonstrate little change in the significant morbidity experienced by patients. Thirty per cent of patients participating in the "Asthma Insights and Reality in Europe" study (AIRE)[5] reported asthma-related sleep disturbance at least once a week. Over half of the adults had daytime symptoms at least once a week and 28% required urgent health care for uncontrolled asthma during the previous 12 months (Figure 1).

Incidence

The range of asthma incidence is wide, both across and within age groups. In young children the range is 4–39% and in older children 1–29%. In adults the range is 1–11%.

Activity limitation due to asthma								
Activity (% limitation)	AIRE Total	UK	France	Germany	The Netherlands	Sweden	Spain	Italy
	2803	400	402	400	400	400	401	400
Sports and recreation	42	29	61	66	41	41	59	41
Normal physical activity	32	26	43	42	28	28	41	37
Choice of jobs or careers	23	16	32	31	24	23	29	28
Social activities	22	17	24	43	27	25	20	19
Sleeping	35	26	53	46	32	24	42	40
Lifestyle	29	19	48	45	32	25	32	30
Housekeeping chores	27	19	46	40	27	17	28	30
NET: any of these	63	49	86	85	68	61	72	71

Figure 1. AIRE study of activity limitation due to asthma. *Source*: AIRE resources page (www.asthma.ac.psiweb.com/index.html). Image courtesy of Prof. Marc Humbert, Service de Pneumologie et Réanimation Respiratoire, Clinique de l'Asthme, Hopital Antoine-Béclère, Université Paris Sud, Clamart, France.

There are differences between males and females, with a higher incidence in young male children and a tendency towards greater number of female older children and adults.

Prevalence

Many studies have examined the prevalence of asthma, most recently the European Community Respiratory Health Survey (ECRHS)[6] and the International Study of Asthma and Allergies in Childhood (ISAAC).[7]

According to the World Health Organization (WHO) estimate in 2000, between 100 and 150 million people worldwide have asthma.

The world map depicted in Figure 2 indicates a greater prevalence of asthma in western countries.[8] The average prevalence rate for asthma in Western Europe is greater in children (13%) than adults (8.4%).[9] There has been a rise in prevalence over the past 15 years of somewhere between 2% and 4%. The reasons for this increase are unclear. However, prevalence is increasing in developing countries; various theories have been suggested to explain this rise (see Figure 3 and Table 1).

Although the prevalence is high in children, most notably in infants, longitudinal studies show that in many cases childhood asthma enters a remission period in adulthood. Where there is coexistent atopy or female gender, the asthma is more likely to persist. If the asthma is more severe

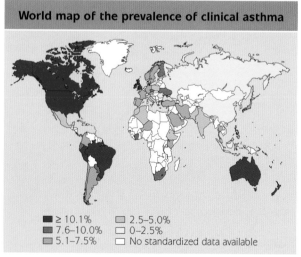

Figure 2. World map of the prevalence of clinical asthma. Image courtesy of Prof. Marc Humbert, Service de Pneumologie et Réanimation Respiratoire, Clinique de l'Asthme, Hopital Antoine-Béclère, Université Paris Sud, Clamart, France.

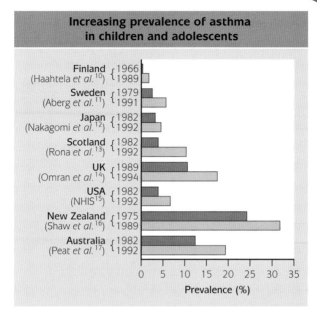

Figure 3. Increased prevalence of asthma in children and adolescents. *Source*: adapted from *Global Strategy for Asthma Management and Prevention*, NIH handbook online (www.ginasthma.com/). Image courtesy of Prof. Marc Humbert, Service de Pneumologie et Réanimation Respiratoire, Clinique de l'Asthme, Hopital Antoine-Béclère, Université Paris Sud, Clamart, France.

Table 1. Possible reasons for increased prevalence of asthma
An increase in the house dust mite population as a consequence of changing domestic living habits
A decrease in exposure to bacterial pathogens during early childhood
Changes in diet leading to a decrease in dietary antioxidants and an increase in polyunsaturated fats
Increased airborne pollution from diesel emissions

in childhood with a history of reduced lung function and frequent exacerbations, the more likely the disease is to persist into adult life. In a longitudinal study,[18] in people aged from 9 to 26, asthma persisted in the group of females with a history of smoking at age 20. A history of smoking is not necessarily associated with persistent disease, but where the disease does persist it is likely to be more severe in such cases.

Mortality

Although people with asthma suffer from very significant morbidity, the relative death rate from this disease is low. The worldwide mortality rate according to World Health Organization (WHO) data is currently 180,000/year; tragically, the great majority of these asthma deaths are considered to be "avoidable". When comparisons are made between the two world maps of prevalence and deaths (see Figures 2 and 4), it seems that a higher level of asthma deaths occur in countries with a lower diagnostic rate.[8] Taking into account the different health systems and economic climate of different countries, the term "avoidable" is used advisedly. However, it is clear that if internationally agreed standards of asthma care are applied, the death rate from asthma could be very much reduced.[19]

The risk factors for asthma

Various environmental factors have been implicated in the development and expression of asthma, and it is often difficult to distinguish between the causes of the development of asthma and trigger factors. There are the predisposing, causal, contributory and aggravating factors. Predisposing factors such as gender and atopy have been mentioned above. Causal factors include domestic and outdoor environmental factors such as allergens, as well as occupational factors. Contributory factors include respiratory infections, especially in childhood and infancy, low birth weight, exposure to active and passive tobacco smoke, and dietary factors. Aggravating factors include

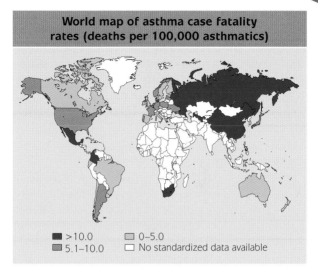

World map of asthma case fatality rates (deaths per 100,000 asthmatics)

■ >10.0   □ 0–5.0
■ 5.1–10.0   □ No standardized data available

Figure 4. World map of asthma deaths. Image courtesy of Prof. Marc Humbert, Service de Pneumologie et Réanimation Respiratoire, Clinique de l'Asthme, Hopital Antoine-Béclère, Université Paris Sud, Clamart, France.

allergens, respiratory infections, physical exercise, weather conditions, food additives and medicines.

The genetics of asthma

Considerable research seeking genetic and environmental links with asthma has concluded that strong elements of heredity influence the onset and outcome of the disease; family history of asthma being one of the most important risk factors,[20] in addition to history of eczema and atopy (positive skin prick tests).[21]

Environmental exposure, intra-uterine[22] and after birth, particularly exposure to maternal smoke, poses significant risks to the child of developing asthma.[23] Ethnic differences in prevalence rates do exist, and while these may be due to problems related to access to care, the precise cause of these variations is unclear.

Viral infections are recognized triggers of asthma; however, it is unclear why some children exhibit wheezing in response to viral infections and others do not. Children who wheeze due to viral infections are more likely to have a past history of atopic eczema and elevated immunoglobulin E (IgE) levels.[24,25] Furthermore, recent studies suggest a link in heredity between the genetic factors for bronchial hyper-responsiveness (BHR) and over-expression of IgE, further to which a chromosome locus for the regulation of IgE has been identified.[1]

Many parents ask whether their child will "grow out of asthma". While there are many studies that conclude that children do not generally "grow out of asthma", it goes into remission, a major research question relates to identification of those whose asthma is likely to persist. Busse and Rosenwasser,[26] in their review, discuss the hypothesis that persistence, i.e. severity of asthma, is related to the balance between production of TH1 (Interferon Gamma or IFγ) versus TH2 (IL-4, IL-5 and IL-13) cytokines, with relative reduction in production of TH1 cytokines favouring persistence of asthma. In a study to predict factors related to persistence or relapse in asthmatic people, Sears et al.[18] followed up a cohort of 613 patients from 9 to 26 years of age. The factors they deemed important were sensitization to house dust mites, airway hyper-responsiveness, female sex, smoking and early age at onset.

Occupational asthma affects about 6% of the asthma population, and factors associated with this condition include the work and climatic environment, as well as genetic factors.[27]

A growing understanding of the genetic factors associated with asthma may increase our understanding of the development and expression of the disease. In addition, this understanding may also lead to greater refining and more specific targeting of the therapeutic treatment of asthma, where, for example, drugs known to be ineffective in the presence of particular polymorphisms could be avoided, and treatment is more specifically targeted to the individual.

The Pathophysiology of Asthma

Asthma is characterized by reversible airway narrowing. This narrowing affects both large and small airways, and is caused by two main elements (see Figure 5): smooth muscle dysfunction and inflammation of the airways. Smooth muscle dysfunction comprises spasm of the bronchial smooth muscle, smooth muscle hyperplasia as a result of persistent spasm and bronchial hyper-responsiveness, causing an increased response to a variety of subsequent stimuli. The inflammation associated with asthma is characterized by oedema, epithelial cell damage and consequent airway remodelling, with thickening of the basement membrane.

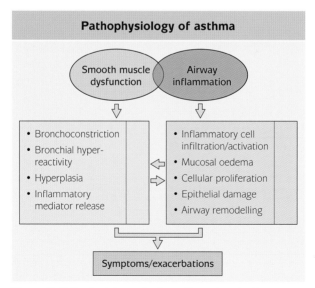

Figure 5. Pathophysiology of asthma. Reproduced with permission from Allen and Hanburys.

Both smooth muscle dysfunction and inflammation are characterized by release of inflammatory mediators and cytokines. Oedema and epithelial cell damage result in the production of excess mucus, which becomes tenacious or sticky due to increased numbers of cells. Some areas of the lung can become under- or hypoventilated due to the obstruction of the airways as a result of the combination of spasm, inflammation and mucus plugging (see Figure 6). The blood continues to flow to the hypoventilated areas, which leads to a ventilation/perfusion mismatch, resulting

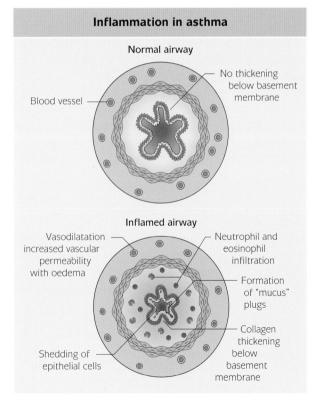

Figure 6. Inflammation and airway obstruction in asthma. Reproduced with permission from Allen and Hanburys.

in hypoxaemia with little change in arterial pH or $PaCO_2$. Arterial hypoxaemia is frequently present in moderate to severe attacks of asthma.

Asthma attacks

During an asthma attack patients' hyperventilate, which is an attempt at increasing oxygen levels in the blood that results in a fall in $PaCO_2$. As the attack progresses, the ability of the patient to compensate for the hypoxaemia by hyperventilation of unobstructed areas of the lung is reduced by progressive and more extensive airway narrowing and general fatigue. In severe attacks the arterial hypoxaemia will worsen and, together with a rising $PaCO_2$, leads to respiratory acidosis and respiratory failure.

When testing lung function, a feature of an early attack is a fall in the maximum mid-expiratory flow. As the attack continues, the forced expiratory volume in the first second of expiration (FEV_1) and the forced vital capacity (FVC) both decrease with associated air trapping and a rise in residual volume. This leads to hyperinflation, which in persistent asthma will become a chronic feature. Abnormalities in flow rates may persist for some time after an acute asthma attack has resolved, even in the presence of "normal" lung function tests.

Mechanism of bronchoconstriction

Although the precise mechanism of the bronchoconstrictor element of asthma is not precisely defined, it is thought that an imbalance between β-adrenergic and cholinergic control may be involved. These abnormalities may be under control of cyclic 3',5'-adenosine monophosphate (cAMP)–cyclic 3',5'-guanosine monophosphate (cGMP) systems in tissues such as mast cells and smooth muscle cells. Intracellular levels of cAMP are a prime effector of smooth muscle tone. They are also associated with inhibition of IgE-related release of chemical mediators, such as histamine, which are involved in the initiation of bronchoconstriction as well as the initiation of the inflammatory cascade.

Inflammatory cascade

The inflammatory cascade is complex and comprises many interacting elements. The breakdown of the epithelial cell membrane leads not only to the release of cytokines and arachidonic acid, the release of arachidonic acid also leads to the further release of leukotrienes and prostaglandins. Inflammatory mediators released by mast cells, eosinophils, lymphocytes and macrophages include histamine, proteins and cytokines. The release of these pro-inflammatory agents continues and reinforces the inflammatory process, leading to a rapidly worsening airway narrowing characteristic of the acute asthma attack. A highly simplified schema in Figure 7 outlines the inflammatory cascade.

The consequences of inflammation can result in airway dysfunction and permanently altered lung function (see Figure 6). In patients who have died as a result of an acute severe asthma attack, post-mortem findings show the presence of glutinous secretions, which may develop into mucus plugs. These plugs can obstruct both large and small airways. The walls of the bronchi will show significant oedema, with thickening of the subepithelial basement membrane and extensive infiltration with eosinophils. The smooth muscle will also show evidence of hyperplasia.

As the understanding of the smooth muscle dysfunction/inflammatory process involved in asthma has progressed, so therapeutic agents have been developed to counteract the disease.

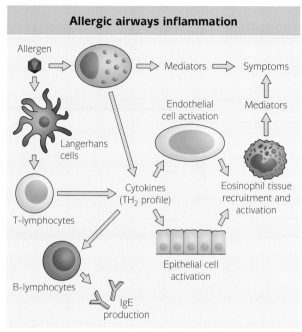

Figure 7. The inflammatory cascade in allergic asthma.

Diagnosis

Introduction

In the last 20 years there has been a considerable reduction in the long delays between the onset of respiratory symptoms and the diagnosis of asthma in children;[28–32] however, many patients are still prescribed asthma medication before a diagnosis is made.[33]

The family doctor or nurse practitioner is usually the first person the patient consults. In primary care, patients present with a variety of symptoms and diseases, which may include extremely vague descriptions of ill health, symptoms specific to particular diseases, as well as acute life-threatening illnesses. These patients present in primary care at all stages of their disease, ranging from those with pre-clinical disease states (i.e. before there are any clear manifestations) to patients manifesting overt advanced, clinically obvious diagnoses.

There is still evidence of delayed diagnosis of asthma, in all spheres of delivery of care. A lack of awareness, by health professionals, of the presenting symptoms of asthma might explain this delay.[34] However, in primary care most health professionals work to a very tight time schedule, often dictated by the numbers of patients under their care. The duration of a patient's appointment with a doctor in primary care varies from country to country and is often as little as 8 minutes. Nurses running dedicated clinics often have more time and are often seeing patients for follow-up. In the case of new consultations, for undiagnosed patients, the doctor or nurse has limited time, during which they have to take a history, examine the patient, administer immediate necessary treatment, prescribe medication, arrange for investigations, make plans for follow-up, and arrange to refer the patient to a specialist. As a result, patients are often treated symptomatically without a clear diagnosis, or before the diagnosis has been confirmed.[9,33]

On the other hand, one of the greatest advantages for the patient in consulting their general practitioner or asthma nurse is the fact that they often get to know one another fairly well and, over time, with cumulative knowledge gained from repeat consultations, an accurate diagnosis is usually made. In this section we describe an approach to diagnosis of asthma and methods of differentiating this condition from other respiratory conditions, particularly chronic obstructive pulmonary disease (COPD), in adults.

Process of diagnosis in primary care

Primary care physicians and nurses are used to working very quickly and therefore, during consultations, adopt a conscious or subliminal process, driven by patients' presenting symptoms, of hypothesis generation and testing (see Figure 8). The symptoms presented result in the generation of a theoretical list of prospective diagnoses; these are either confirmed or eliminated as possibilities by further questioning, examination or investigations. If none of these lead to a firm diagnosis, more hypotheses or lists are generated and the process is repeated. This process of hypothesis generation and testing in primary care may span a number of short consultations, complemented by access to past medical records and knowledge of the family and social background, often involving different health professionals. In contrast, in the hospital setting, the patient often presents with a detailed summary of the medical problem provided by the general practitioner, and then the process of diagnosis involves a comprehensive history, examination and investigation of the patient. This usually occurs during one long out-patient consultation or in-patient stay.

There are major problems related to diagnosis of the common respiratory diseases in primary care. People with asthma, by definition, fluctuate from one extreme to another with respect to their symptoms, lung function and response to medication. As a result, patients may manifest overt signs and symptoms or none at all. In fact, there are even patients who may exhibit no signs or symptoms during an acute attack of asthma.[35] In the case of patients with combined asthma and COPD, who may have demonstrable,

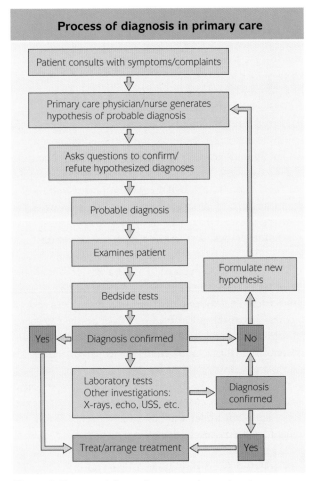

Figure 8. Process of diagnosis – generating and testing hypotheses.

reversible airflow obstruction, this causes difficulty in making a clear diagnosis. Patients with allergic disease may present with features of asthma, adding a further dimension and making it even more difficult to confirm a diagnosis. Lack of facilities for investigating respiratory or allergic diseases in primary care, such as spirometry or skin prick testing equipment, places very heavy reliance on the clinical skills of the primary care health professional.

Mode of presentation

Screening and case finding are two of the population-based processes utilized in diagnosing diseases. The former involves investigating large numbers of people, often asymptomatic, and is very time-consuming, with the possibility of failing to identify many patients with the disease at high cost. Case finding is more targeted and relies on identifying patients with a higher probability of having the disease in question. In primary care diagnosis of respiratory disease, case finding is more realistic, relying on patients presenting with symptoms and signs suggestive of respiratory disease.

Patients present in primary care with complaints or symptoms that may be very specific and provide clear clues to diagnosis; however, this is unusual. In reality, people often present their own diagnoses and interpretation of the symptoms, with a clear expectation that the doctor or nurse will be able to provide curative treatment. The patients' agenda, therefore, may influence and sometimes delay the process of diagnosis. Health professionals need to be fully aware of the different patterns of presentation of patients with asthma, at different stages of their disease. They also need to be aware of the risk of being influenced by patients' perceptions of their problem and making a hasty, incorrect diagnosis when under time pressure. Figures 9 and 10 summarize the process of diagnosis in children and adults.[35]

Symptoms of asthma

Recurrent wheeze, cough, breathlessness and chest tightness, and chest pain are the commonest symptoms suggestive of

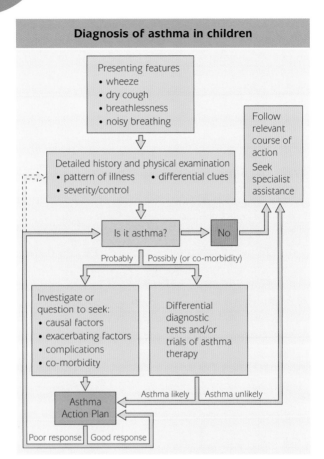

Figure 9. Diagnosis of asthma in children. *Source*: British Thoracic Society/SIGN (www.brit-thoracic.org.uk/sign/index.htm). Reproduced from: British guidelines on the management of asthma. *Thorax* 2003; **58**(Suppl 1): i1–i94.[35]

asthma in children and adults. Initial presentation with one or more of these symptoms may occur at any age (termed late-onset asthma if in adulthood). There are many other causes of these symptoms in childhood (see Figure 11). In trying to establish a diagnosis in children, health professionals often depend on the parent's description of

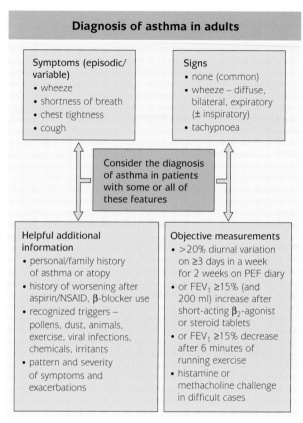

Diagnosis of asthma in adults

Symptoms (episodic/variable)
- wheeze
- shortness of breath
- chest tightness
- cough

Signs
- none (common)
- wheeze – diffuse, bilateral, expiratory (± inspiratory)
- tachypnoea

Consider the diagnosis of asthma in patients with some or all of these features

Helpful additional information
- personal/family history of asthma or atopy
- history of worsening after aspirin/NSAID, β-blocker use
- recognized triggers – pollens, dust, animals, exercise, viral infections, chemicals, irritants
- pattern and severity of symptoms and exacerbations

Objective measurements
- >20% diurnal variation on ≥3 days in a week for 2 weeks on PEF diary
- or FEV_1 ≥15% (and 200 ml) increase after short-acting $β_2$-agonist or steroid tablets
- or FEV_1 ≥15% decrease after 6 minutes of running exercise
- histamine or methacholine challenge in difficult cases

Figure 10. Diagnosis of asthma in adults. *Source*: British Thoracic Society/SIGN (www.brit-thoracic.org.uk/sign/index.htm). Reproduced from: British guidelines on the management of asthma. *Thorax* 2003; **58**(Suppl 1): i1–i94.[35]

symptoms. However, some parents are unclear what wheeze sounds like, and mistake noisy breathing from upper airway secretions or even stridor for wheeze. Recurrent cough, especially at night or with exercise, is reported more commonly than wheeze, especially in preschool asthmatic children. In adults, cardiac or respiratory problems (such as cardiac failure or recurrent pulmonary emboli), or patients with dysfunctional breathing, may present with

Clues to alternative diagnoses in wheezy children

Clinical clue	Possible diagnosis
Perinatal and family history	
• symptoms present from birth or perinatal lung problem	• cystic fibrosis, chronic lung disease, ciliary dyskinesia, developmental anomaly
• family history of unusual chest disease	• cystic fibrosis, developmental anomaly, neuromuscular disorder
• severe upper respiratory tract disease	• defect of host defence

Figure 11. Clues to alternative diagnoses in children. *Source*: British Thoracic Society/SIGN (www.brit-thoracic.org.uk/sign/index.htm). Reproduced from: British guidelines on the management of asthma. *Thorax* 2003; **58**(Suppl 1): i1–i94.[35]

recurrent respiratory symptoms and mimic asthma (see Figure 12). In the UK, patients records follow them from doctor to doctor, providing a continuous record of medical consultations (and hospital attendances), and therefore perusal of the past medical record, combined with a detailed history, may often provide additional evidence to support a diagnosis of asthma.[31,34,36,37] The General Practice Airways Group has developed a label that can be inserted in the patients' record to denote the method of diagnosis of asthma (see Figure 13).

The diagnosis of asthma is supported by a history that the symptoms are precipitated by particular trigger factors (see Table 2). Viral upper respiratory tract infections in the younger child, and exercise in the older child, are the most common and easily recognized triggers in childhood. Factors in older children and adults include: viral infections, emotional upset or excitement, sudden changes in

Figure 12. Differential diagnosis of asthma. Reproduced with permission from the International Primary Care Airways Group (IPAG). IPAG guidelines document in press.

Differential diagnosis of asthma – causes of breathlessness, wheezing or coughing

Children	Adults
Virus-associated wheeze (VAW) **Upper airway disease** • adenotonsillar hypertrophy • rhinosinusitus • postnasal drip **Congenital structural bronchial disease** • complete cartilage rings • cysts • webs **Bronchial tracheal compression** • vascular rings and sling • enlarged cardiac chamber • lymphnodes enlarged by TB or lymphoma **Endobronchial disease** • foreign body • tumour **Oesophageal/swallowing problems** • reflux • incoordinate swallow • laryngeal cleft • tracheo-oesophageal fistula **Causes of pulmonary suppuration** • cystic fibrosis • primary ciliary dyskinesia • systemic immunodeficiency **Miscellaneous** • bronchiectasis • bronchopulmonary dysplasia • tracheomalacia • tuberculosis • pulmonary oedema	**Lung disease** Acute: • pulmonary embolism • pleural effusions • atelectasis collapse Chronic: • bronchiectasis • COPD • malignancy • sarcoidosis • tuberculosis • fibrosing/allergic alveolitis • eosinophilic pneumonia • chest wall deformity • asbestosis **Heart disease** Acute: • myocardial infarction - cardiac rhythm disturbance - left ventricular failure Chronic: • chronic heart failure • valve disease • cardiomyopathy Foreign body aspiration **Systemic disorders – breathlessness** • anaemia • obesity • hyperthyroidism **Dysfunctional breathing** Consider if: • symptoms disproportionate to objective signs • severe symptoms with normal lung function • upper chest rather than diaphragmatic breathing • "unusual" symptom patterns

Clues to alternative diagnoses in wheezy children

Asthma diagnosis (three ticks confirm a diagnosis of asthma)		
Yes	√ A typical history	Variable symptoms of wheeze, cough, shortness of breath, chest tightness, PMH of FH of atopy
Yes	√ 20% variability	Peak flow diary showing: 20% diurnal variation 20% reduction after trigger 20% response to treatment
Yes	√ Response to treatment	Symptomatic response to β_2-agonist, oral/inhaled steroid
Asthma: diagnosed/not diagnosed/suspected		

Figure 13. Diagnosis of asthma. *Source:* GPIAG opinion sheets (www.gpiag.org).[38] Reproduced with permission from Dr Mark Levy, Editor GPIAG.

Table 2. Trigger factors for asthma

Colds and viral infections

Pets

Exercise

Allergen exposure, e.g. house dust mites, pollen

Tobacco smoke

Emotional upset

Chemical irritants

Fumes

Cold air

Occupational exposure

Medications: e.g. β-blockers and NSAIDs

temperature or humidity, exposure to common allergens such as cats, dogs or grass pollens, and the inhalation of chemical irritants such as cigarette smoke or domestic aerosols.

Elderly patients pose particular diagnostic and therapeutic problems in asthma because there are often other concomitant diseases present. Asthma in older people is under-diagnosed,[39,40] sometimes misdiagnosed,[41] and therefore undertreated. In some elderly patients the respiratory symptoms are non-specific; physical examination may be unhelpful and the ability to do peak expiratory flow (PEF) readings impaired. In these circumstances spirometry may be more helpful or, failing this, the response to a trial of therapy.

Confirming the diagnosis of asthma and chronic obstructive pulmonary disease (COPD)

Asthma can be diagnosed on the basis of the medical history in the majority of patients (see Table 3). Ideally, this diagnosis should be confirmed using objective measurements. In older adults, particularly those with a history of smoking, asthma does need to be differentiated from COPD.

Chronic obstructive pulmonary disease is defined as an obstructive airways disorder which is largely irreversible

Table 3. Clues to diagnosis of asthma

Recurrent consultations for respiratory symptoms:
- Cough
- Wheeze
- Difficulty in breathing

"Colds" that don't clear up or prolonged cough following a viral infection

Variability of symptoms

Variability of symptoms, signs and lung function

May be normal or asymptomatic between attacks

Past history of allergy, eczema, atopy or allergic rhinitis

Family history of asthma, allergy, eczema, atopy or allergic rhinitis (see definition below). While the medical history is helpful in this regard, the diagnosis should ideally be confirmed with spirometry testing. COPD is diagnosed if the FEV_1/FVC ratio is below 70% and the severity is classified according to the % Predicted FEV_1 (see below). Demonstration of fixed (irreversible) or reversible airflow obstruction helps to confirm the diagnosis of COPD and asthma respectively. However, there is considerable controversy regarding the extent to which reversibility occurs in COPD. Some patients with COPD do demonstrate reversibility of airflow obstruction: are these patients actually suffering from asthma?

Definition of COPD[42]

"Chronic obstructive pulmonary disease (COPD) is a disease state characterized by airflow limitation that is not fully reversible. The airflow limitation is usually both progressive and associated with an abnormal inflammatory response of the lungs to noxious particles or gases."

Peak expiratory flow (PEF)

Repeated measurement of PEF is used to demonstrate variable airflow obstruction. The best of three measurements is taken either before and after a bronchodilator or after exercise (in children), or over a period of time by using a diary chart. There are a number of methods for calculating PEF variability; the one used most widely is the amplitude (maximum – minimum) as a percentage of the maximum, as shown in Table 4, where amplitude is the difference between readings from morning to evening, from day to day, or before and after medication or exercise.

A change in PEF of 20% is usually accepted as confirmation of the diagnosis of asthma.[35] PEF meters may vary in accuracy, and therefore variability of PEF readings using different meters, even of the same type, may reach 20% (UK regulations allow for ±10% variation from the

Table 4. Method for calculating peak expiratory flow variability

$$\text{PEF variability} = \frac{\text{Maximum PEF} - \text{Minimum PEF}}{\text{Maximum PEF}} \times 100$$

gold standard). In addition, the use of different scales for PEF meters in various countries adds to the confusion if patients have acquired meters from other countries. Predicted PEF values also vary between meters, and comparisons should be made to reference charts based on height, sex and ethnicity, which may not be available for each population group. For these reasons, patients should have their own meter and PEF measurements are ideally compared to the patient's own previous best measurements, using the same peak flow meter. Ideally, PEF should be measured first thing in the morning, when values are usually at their lowest, and in the afternoon, when they are usually at their highest.

Spirometry

Spirometry is regarded as more reliable and repeatable than PEF, and is considered essential in diagnosing COPD and differentiating this disease from restrictive respiratory diseases. The forced expiratory volume in 1 second (FEV_1), forced vital capacity (FVC) and the ratio of the two (FEV_1/FVC) are used most frequently.

FEV_1/FVC below 70% confirms the diagnosis of airflow obstruction,[42] which together with FEV_1 measurements (below 80% predicted), are used to grade severity of COPD. These vary between guidelines. A variation in FEV_1 of over 15% is accepted for confirmation of a diagnosis of asthma, although there is considerable debate on this matter.

Prevention of Asthma and Allergen Avoidance

Can asthma be prevented? Does it persist? These are two of the commonest questions asked by patients and parents. The two areas where intervention has proved effective in preventing asthma development or deterioration are in the case of exposure to occupational factors or aspirin-induced asthma. These are discussed briefly later in this book (see pp. 106 and 109). Asthma prevention should logically begin in infancy or even pre-conception, and there has been a considerable amount of research in this area. Some researchers have focused on the natural history of the disease through longitudinal follow-up of children,[43] while others have studied avoidance of known associated allergens of asthma, such as parental smoking and exposure to house dust mites. For example, one study concluded that the use of allergen-impermeable covers, as a single intervention for the avoidance of exposure to dust mite allergen, seems clinically ineffective in adults with asthma.[44] Another group of studies investigated whether prophylactic drug therapy has helped prevent the development of asthma. The ETAC study of infants with atopic dermatitis, which is a common precursor of asthma, concluded that cetirizine compared with placebo delayed or, in some cases, prevented the development of asthma in some infants.[45] This study also highlights risk factors for asthma in infants with atopic dermatitis, and indicates that early and persistent aeroallergen sensitization confers a higher risk than later development of sensitivity. In the future, we may see studies involving genetic manipulation and intervention.

A recent longitudinal study by Malcolm Sears and colleagues[18] has investigated the factors which lead to persistence and relapse of the disease. They collected data on 613 patients over a period of 26 years; data collected were derived from questionnaires, pulmonary function tests, bronchial challenge testing and allergy testing. As others have found, these researchers reported that patients who persist with asthma often start wheezing earlier compared with those who remit. Thirteen per cent of patients who had "grown out of their asthma" had relapsed before their 26th birthday; however, this study has demonstrated that those who later relapsed had started suffering from their symptoms earlier. Martinez concludes from this that "These findings provide strong support for the contention that environmental factors, acting during early life and interacting with specific 'asthma genes', are crucial for the development of the chronic, persistent form of the disease."[43] Females were more likely to persist with wheezing than males, as were patients with house dust mite sensitization, particularly if they smoked at age 21. Maternal smoking during pregnancy and infancy has been associated with impaired lung growth and reduced lung function. A meta-analysis has estimated that exposure to tobacco smoke up to the age of 6 years increases the risk of developing asthma by 37% and after the age of 6 by 13%.[46]

Viral infections play a role in triggering asthma exacerbations; they have also been implicated as a cause or rather that they might prevent the development of asthma. The "hygiene hypothesis", which was introduced by Strachan,[47] suggested that reduction in exposure to virus infections was responsible for increased clinical symptoms due to allergic disease. This was based on the theory that virus infections protect children from developing allergic disease. This is a subject of current debate and no doubt research will provide more data for the future.

A number of factors, both genetic and environmental, play a part in the development of asthma or trigger asthma exacerbations. Some of these can be avoided, particularly for primary prevention and exacerbations (see Table 5).

Table 5. Factors that play a role in the development of asthma
Environmental risk factors
Active smoking
Passive smoking
Occupational exposure
Indoor air pollutants, e.g. house dust mites
Outdoor air pollutants, e.g. sulphur dioxide
Meteorological conditions
Allergens
Diet
Socio-economic status
Endogenous risk factors
Genetics
Sex
Familial history
Low birth weight
Respiratory infections

Management of Asthma

Assessment and monitoring

Patients with asthma may be assessed at various intervals and on specific occasions (see Table 6). These could include: a consultation, with the aim of confirming asthma following initial suspicion of the diagnosis; perhaps to review diary cards; and lung function responses to a trial of therapy. Patients may consult for routine follow-up to ascertain whether their medication needs to be altered by "stepping up or stepping down". Many patients with asthma suffer from ongoing symptoms without realizing that optimal management of their condition could alleviate these. They "put up with" reduced quality of life. Therefore, one of the main aims of routine monitoring is to identify any troublesome symptoms, to try and establish the root cause of these, and to advise on appropriate measures to rectify the situation. Consultations may be at the request of the doctor or nurse if they notice that excess prescriptions are being ordered, indicating possible poor asthma control. Similarly, the local pharmacist may refer patients who consult them frequently for symptomatic relief of respiratory

Table 6. Purpose for assessment and monitoring consultations
Confirming the diagnosis (review diary cards and lung function responses to a trial of therapy)
Routine follow-up
Request of the doctor or nurse (for perceived poor asthma control)
Request of other health professionals (e.g. pharmacist, secondary care, district nurse)
Follow-up for acute asthma exacerbations

Table 7. Six-step approach to monitoring asthma patients

i	Ascertain the patient's current treatment and compliance
ii	Establish whether the patient has any symptoms and the relevant trigger factors
iii	Determine whether the patient's lung function is satisfactory
iv	Check inhaler technique
v	Advise on medication: step-up, step-down, change medication or device
vi	Arrange to review the patient at an appropriate interval

Reproduced from Levy ML *et al.* A randomized controlled evaluation of specialist nurse education following accident and emergency department attendance for acute asthma. *Respir Med* 2000; **94**(9): 900–908[48] with permission from Elsevier Limited.

symptoms. Finally, and perhaps most importantly, consultations may follow acute asthma exacerbations. The principles underlying the health professionals' approach to these consultations are similar and are summarized in an approach which was effective in a randomized controlled study involving follow-up of patients after an asthma attack prompting a hospital attendance.[48]

We advocate a "six-step approach" in monitoring patients (see Table 7),[48] as well as reconsidering the accuracy of the diagnosis at each consultation, until finally confirmed, and also suggest that the method of diagnosis is recorded in the medical record (see Figure 13). Many patients attend for "asthma review" without ever having had the diagnosis confirmed. The major disadvantage for these patients is that they are often treated inappropriately, for example with antibiotics, where they may actually need anti-asthma treatment. The asthma "review" consultation, therefore, could serve to both confirm the diagnosis as well as to establish the level of asthma control, followed by appropriate intervention.

Classification of severity			
	Classify severity Clinical Features Before Treatment		
	Symptoms	Nocturnal symptoms	FEV$_1$ or PEF
STEP 4 Severe Persistent	Continuous Limited physical activity	Frequent	≤60% predicted Variability >30%
STEP 3 Moderate Persistent	Daily Attacks affect activity	>1 time a week	60–80% predicted Variability >30%
STEP 2 Mild Persistent	>1 time a week but <1 time a day	>2 times a month	≥80% predicted Variability 20–30%
STEP 1 Intermittent	<1 time a week Asymptomatic and normal PEF between attacks	≤2 times a month	≥80% predicted Variability <20%

The presence of one feature of severity is sufficient to place patient in that category

Figure 14. GINA stepwise classification of asthma severity.
Source: www.ginasthma.com.

i. Ascertain the patient's current treatment and compliance

At the start of the consultation, it is helpful to ascertain what medication the patient is actually taking and to record this, perhaps according to the stepwise method in use according to local guidelines. Recording the asthma "steps"[35,49] (see Figures 14, 17–19) is helpful in assessment as well as management decisions on the patient. The fact that someone is prescribed certain medication does not necessarily mean this medication has been dispensed by the pharmacist, or is actually being taken (see p. 94).

ii. Establish whether the patient has any symptoms and their relevant trigger factors

It is not sufficient to simply ask patients whether their asthma "is OK", or to say "how is your asthma?" Many patients will simply say they are fine, without realizing their quality of life could be much better. Specific leading questions such as those advocated by the SIGN/BTS guidelines (see Table 8), specific enquiry about trigger factors (see Table 2) or, perhaps, use of validated quality-of-life questionnaires[50-54] could be used during consultations to establish whether patients' asthma is controlled. Furthermore, specific enquiry regarding factors that triggered these symptoms may help in guiding advice on prevention of future attacks and poor asthma control.

The use of diary cards can also assist in decisions and advice given at assessment and monitoring consultations (see Figures 15 and 16). Recording daily symptoms, night waking and the frequency of use of reliever medication helps both the patient and health professional. Being more aware of the daily consequences of asthma may influence the need for remedial action. Many patients attending for routine asthma review exhibit features of uncontrolled asthma and an astute health professional may be able to avert an attack by advising accordingly. In particular, it is important to determine how frequently reliever medication is used and whether this is having its usual effect; failure of patients to respond in their usual way to reliever medication is a well-recognized danger sign of asthma (see Table 9).

iii. Determine whether the patient's lung function is satisfactory

A PEF diary kept for a week or two preceding the review appointment is extremely helpful in determining asthma control. Variability over 20% indicates inadequate control requiring intervention, either by changing inhaler device or medication as appropriate. The use of a diary in this way also helps to reinforce objective measurement of lung function by the patient, a feature identified as lacking in

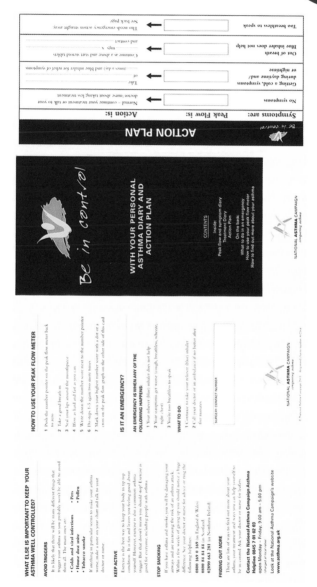

Figure 15. National Asthma Campaign self-management plan. Reproduced with permission from the UK National Asthma Campaign.[79]

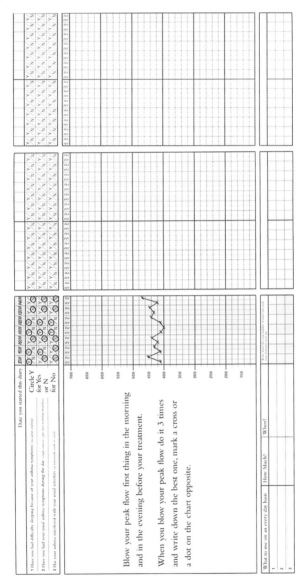

Figure 16. National Asthma Campaign peak flow diary chart. Reproduced with permission from the UK National Asthma Campaign.[79]

Table 8. The Royal College of Physicians (RCP) "three questions"[35,55]

(1) In the last week/month:

Have you had difficulty sleeping because of your asthma symptoms (including cough)?

(2) In the last week/month:

Have you had your usual asthma symptoms during the day (cough, wheeze, chest tightness or breathlessness)?

(3) In the last week/month:

Has your asthma interfered with your usual activities (e.g. housework, work/school, etc.)?

Table 9. Monitoring response to reliever medication – danger signs

β_2-Agonist bronchodilators (e.g. salbutamol, terbutaline) should provide quick relief of symptoms

The relief should last at least 4 hours

recent confidential enquiries into the circumstances surrounding asthma deaths.[3,56] In the consultation, measurement of PEF before and after bronchodilator use, may help to establish PEF variability, and also to reinforce the value of taking these measurements to the patient. Spirometry is indicated in those adults over 40 with a smoking history and respiratory symptoms. Some patients, over 40 years old, being treated for "asthma" may actually have COPD or mixed asthma and COPD, and confirmation of this diagnosis will help direct the future management of these patients.

Table 10. Inhaler device technique scoring method
Adequate preparation of the device
Correct positioning of head and neck
Adequate inhalation technique
Breath holding for 10 seconds

iv. Check inhaler technique (see p. 71)

A simple scoring system may be used to check inhaler technique and to decide whether to prescribe a different device (see Table 10). It is clearly wasteful to prescribe medication that the patients either cannot or will not use for various reasons.

v. Advise on medication: step-up, step-down, change medication or device (see p. 45)

Decisions at this stage of the consultation will depend upon the outcome of the preceding four steps. The presence of symptoms, impaired quality of life and variation in lung function would indicate the need for adjusting medication, provided of course that the diagnosis of asthma is correct. In the authors' experience, it is not uncommon for patients with alternative diagnoses to be treated for "asthma" for many years. Therefore, it would be prudent, before changing device or adding therapy, to exclude other diagnoses such as bronchiectasis, in patients whose "asthma" is uncontrolled despite adequate management. If the inhaler technique was inadequate, a change of device or addition of a spacer is indicated. If not, then either increasing current medication or addition of new medication (stepping up) is appropriate. However, if the patient's asthma is well controlled, then it would be quite appropriate to advise a reduction in medication (stepping down). Through recording the steps at the beginning and the end of the consultation, medical audit is facilitated by providing data that can be analysed to assess health professionals' management decisions during asthma consultations.[48]

vi. Arrange to review the patient at an appropriate interval

The time interval until the next review appointment will be determined by the outcome of the review consultation. Patients with uncontrolled asthma, who have been advised a change in medication, should be seen sooner. Use of a PEF diary is also advisable in the event that patients' medication was either stepped up or down during this consultation.

Therapeutic management

The modern therapeutic management of asthma has evolved from the time when there was almost complete reliance on reliever medications to nowadays, where the emphasis is centred on controlling the disease and reducing the need for therapy providing relief from acute symptoms.

The model of modern treatment is expressed in the recent British Guidelines on Asthma Management (BGAM), published in *Thorax* in 2003.[35] The model follows previous iterations of British asthma guidelines in adopting a stepwise system of management. In this latest version, the patient is initiated on a level and choice of medication considered appropriate for their asthma and its mode of presentation. Thereafter, medication is adjusted with the increase or reduction of therapy, and the addition or removal of individual medications (see Figures 17–19). The international GINA (Global Initiative on Asthma) guidelines follow the same stepwise management (see Figure 14), but patients are placed in categories of degrees of severity rather than in therapeutic groups as in the BGAM.

Asthma is a condition that can be controlled by medications as well as avoidance of trigger factors (see p. 34). The aims of pharmacological management are assessed by the following standards:

- Minimal symptoms during day and night.
- Minimal need for reliever medications.
- No exacerbations.

Summary of stepwise management in adults

STEP 5: Continuous or frequent use of oral steroids

Use daily steroid tablet in lowest dose providing adequate control

Maintain high-dose inhaled steroid at 2000 mcg/day*

Consider other treatments to minimize the use of steroid tablets

Refer patient for specialist care

STEP 4: Persistent poor control

Consider trials of:
- increasing inhaled steroid up to 2000mcg/day*
- addition of a fourth drug, e.g. leukotriene receptor antagonist, SR theophylline, β_2-agonist tablet

STEP 3: Add-on therapy

1. Add inhaled long-acting β_2-agonist (LABA)
2. Assess control of asthma:
- **good response to LABA** – continue LABA
- **benefit from LABA** but control still inadequate – continue LABA and increase inhaled steroid dose to 800 mcg/day* (if not already on this dose)
- **no response to LABA** – stop LABA and increase inhaled steroid to 800 mcg/day*. If control still inadequate, institute trial of other therapies (e.g. leukotriene receptor antagonist or SR theophylline)

STEP 2: Regular preventer therapy

Add inhaled steroid, 200–800 mcg/day*

400 mcg is an appropriate starting dose for many patients

Start at dose of inhaled steroid appropriate to severity of disease

STEP 1: Mild intermittent asthma

Inhaled short-acting β_2-agonist as required

*BDP or equivalent

- No limit of physical activity.
- Normal lung function (FEV_1 and/or PEF >80% predicted or best).[35]

β_2-Agonist bronchodilators

These drugs, the β-sympathomimetics, are synthetic developments of naturally occurring noradrenaline. They act upon the β-receptors causing, in the airways, the relaxation of bronchial smooth muscle. The β-receptors are members of a family of G-protein-coupled receptors – a group of seven transmembrane receptors. The G-protein consists of three subunits, α, β and γ. When the β_2-agonist bronchodilator attaches to the receptor, the subunit splits off and leads to the production of cyclic adenosine monophosphate (cAMP). This mediates the β_2-agonist effects of the drug.

The β_2-agonist bronchodilators are the main class of bronchodilator for the management of asthma. Their development has resulted from a search for drugs that have the bronchodilator effect of the drug class, with minimization of the unwanted effects such as muscle tremor and tachycardia. β_2-Agonist bronchodilators are classified according to the onset and duration of action. Short-acting β_2-agonist bronchodilators such as salbutamol and terbutaline have a 2- to 4-hour bronchodilator effect and are used for short-term relief with symptomatic asthma. There is no evidence of any detrimental effect from using these short-acting bronchodilators on a regular basis, as they do not have any significant detrimental effect.

Figure 17. Stepwise management of adults. *Source*: British Thoracic Society/SIGN (www.brit-thoracic.org.uk/sign/index.htm). Reproduced from: British guidelines on the management of asthma. *Thorax* 2003; **58**(Suppl 1): i1–i94.[35]

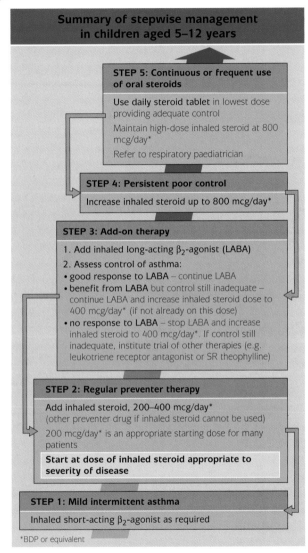

Summary of stepwise management in children aged 5–12 years

STEP 5: Continuous or frequent use of oral steroids

Use daily steroid tablet in lowest dose providing adequate control

Maintain high-dose inhaled steroid at 800 mcg/day*

Refer to respiratory paediatrician

STEP 4: Persistent poor control

Increase inhaled steroid up to 800 mcg/day*

STEP 3: Add-on therapy

1. Add inhaled long-acting β_2-agonist (LABA)
2. Assess control of asthma:
   - good response to LABA – continue LABA
   - benefit from LABA but control still inadequate – continue LABA and increase inhaled steroid dose to 400 mcg/day* (if not already on this dose)
   - no response to LABA – stop LABA and increase inhaled steroid to 400 mcg/day*. If control still inadequate, institute trial of other therapies (e.g. leukotriene receptor antagonist or SR theophylline)

STEP 2: Regular preventer therapy

Add inhaled steroid, 200–400 mcg/day*
(other preventer drug if inhaled steroid cannot be used)

200 mcg/day* is an appropriate starting dose for many patients

Start at dose of inhaled steroid appropriate to severity of disease

STEP 1: Mild intermittent asthma

Inhaled short-acting β_2-agonist as required

*BDP or equivalent

Figure 18. Stepwise management of children 5–12 years old. *Source*: British Thoracic Society/SIGN (www.brit-thoracic.org.uk/sign/index.htm). Reproduced from: British guidelines on the management of asthma. *Thorax* 2003; **58**(Suppl 1): i1–i94.[35]

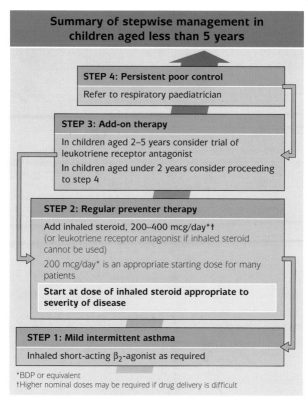

Summary of stepwise management in children aged less than 5 years

STEP 4: Persistent poor control

Refer to respiratory paediatrician

STEP 3: Add-on therapy

In children aged 2–5 years consider trial of leukotriene receptor antagonist

In children aged under 2 years consider proceeding to step 4

STEP 2: Regular preventer therapy

Add inhaled steroid, 200–400 mcg/day*† (or leukotriene receptor antagonist if inhaled steroid cannot be used)

200 mcg/day* is an appropriate starting dose for many patients

Start at dose of inhaled steroid appropriate to severity of disease

STEP 1: Mild intermittent asthma

Inhaled short-acting β_2-agonist as required

*BDP or equivalent
†Higher nominal doses may be required if drug delivery is difficult

Figure 19. Stepwise management of children under 5 years old. *Source*: British Thoracic Society/SIGN (www.brit-thoracic.org.uk/sign/index.htm). Reproduced from: British guidelines on the management of asthma. *Thorax* 2003; **58**(Suppl 1): i1–i94.[35]

The need for regular use of these drugs by the patient suggests uncontrolled asthma.

Long-acting β_2-agonist bronchodilators such as salmeterol and formoterol have a 9- to 12-hour duration of action. They are used as an add-on therapy to inhaled corticosteroid therapy to improve symptom control, improve lung function and reduce exacerbations.

Both short- and long-acting β_2-agonists inhibit the acute early response phase to allergens.

Corticosteroids

Inhaled corticosteroids are the mainstay for the regular treatment of chronic asthma. They have a proven efficacy and a lower potential for systemic side-effects than oral corticosteroids. Several guidelines have been developed worldwide, and they are consistent in their agreement on the use of inhaled corticosteroids in the management of symptomatic asthma (see Table 11).

When inhaled, the molecules of corticosteroids pass through the cell membrane of the airway epithelial cells. Once in the cytoplasm, they conjugate with the corticosteroid receptors, causing the heat-shock proteins (the "chaperone" proteins) to disassociate from the corticosteroid receptors. The corticosteroid/corticosteroid receptor complexes then come together in pairs to form dimers, and in this form pass into the nucleus by translocation, where they attach to specific regions of the DNA. This results in gene transcription, with consequent

Table 11. International asthma guidelines	
British Thoracic Society/ Scottish Intercollegiate Guidelines Network (BTS/SIGN)	www.brit-thoracic.org. uk/docs/SIGN63.PDF
Global Initiative for Asthma (GINA)	www.ginasthma.com/
National Institutes of Health (NIH)	www.nhlbi.nih.gov/new/ press/02-06-10.htm
New Zealand Asthma Guidelines	www.asthmanz.co.nz/
Canadian Asthma Guidelines	www.asthmaguidelines. com/home.html

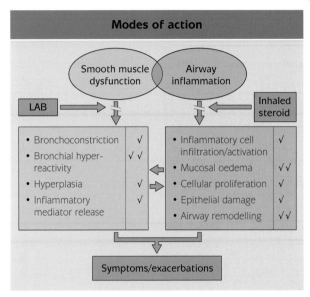

Figure 20. Modes of action of asthma drugs. Reproduced with permission from Allen and Hanburys.

increase in transcription of anti-inflammatory proteins and suppressed transcription of pro-inflammatory genes. In addition, there is also an increase in the synthesis of the β_2-adrenoreceptors.

A number of different inhaled corticosteroids are available, including beclomethasone dipropionate (BDP), budesonide (BUD), fluticasone propionate (FP) and, more recently, mometasone furoate (MF) and ciclesonide (currently applying for license at time of going to press).

Inhaled corticosteroids reduce airway inflammation, reduce airway hyper-responsiveness, improve airflow obstruction and consequently reduce the symptoms of asthma (see Figure 20).[57,58] These findings have led to the use of inhaled corticosteroids as the initial treatment of choice for infants, children and adults with persistent symptoms of asthma. All inhaled corticosteroids differ in potency and bioavailability, and the dose administered should be appropriate to the disease severity and as recommended in the relevant guidelines (see Figure 18).

Oral and injectable corticosteroids are reserved for the management of unremitting severe asthma, or in the short term for acute exacerbations of asthma or as part of a reversibility test to assess response to airflow obstruction.

Combined inhaled corticosteroids and long-acting β_2-agonist bronchodilators, available in one inhaler delivery device, have been developed. In addition to the clinical benefits[59,60] of these two groups of drugs, their combination in one device has the potential to simplify treatment regimes, reduce prescription costs and possibly improve compliance.

Leukotriene receptor antagonists

As opposed to the inhaled corticosteroids, which act on a variety of sites within the inflammatory cascade, the leukotriene receptor antagonists (LTRAs), as their name suggests, block leukotriene receptors. Leukotrienes are one of the major inflammatory modulators in the arachidonic cascade. For those whose asthma is particularly modulated by leukotrienes (probably 20–30% of the asthmatic population), leukotriene receptor antagonists have proved to be effective in controlling asthma. One of their advantages is that they are given orally.

Cromones

The use of inhaled cromones for asthma has reduced recently. A recent systematic review of sodium cromoglycate concluded that there were no proven advantages over placebo. Nedocromil is little used and, as for sodium cromoglycate, there is little evidence to support its clinical effectiveness.

Theophyllines

These drugs are phosphodiasterase inhibitors and act as bronchodilators, but are also thought to have some anti-inflammatory effect in low doses. Their bronchodilator effect is less than that of the β_2-agonist bronchodilators, but may have some additive effect if taken in conjunction.

Their use has declined over the past 10 years as the use of inhaled β_2-agonist bronchodilators has increased. They are taken orally or by injection. They have a narrow therapeutic window, and their unpleasant side-effects (nausea, arrhythmias and headaches) have contributed to their decline. These drugs are recommended for use at step 3[35,49] and step 4 if other medication is not relieving the patient's symptoms.[35,49] They are still used intravenously in the management of acute severe asthma.

Magnesium

Recent studies have suggested a place for the use of intravenous magnesium sulphate under direction of a specialist in a hospital setting. The drug is administered as a single-dose bolus in acute severe asthma, and has a bronchodilator effect.

Oxygen

In acute severe asthma, patients become hypoxic, and therefore oxygen has a key role in all cases of acute severe asthma. Where available, it should be used to drive a nebulizer containing bronchodilator medication. A flow rate of 6 litres/minute is required for effective nebulization and therefore, if cylinder oxygen is used, this should have a high-flow regulator fitted. If a high-flow regulator is not available, oxygen should still be administered in addition to the nebulized therapy (see p. 58).

Omalizumab

Anti-IgE monoclonal antibody therapies have been developed. As yet they are unavailable in the UK (also see p. 112).

Clinical pathways

As stated earlier, administration of asthma treatment is generally recommended in a stepwise manner. We have referred mainly to the recent British Thoracic Society/SIGN guidelines[35] in the text; however, we have provided figures to illustrate both these and the GINA guidelines. The scope of this book has prevented us from summarizing other national guidelines; however, these may be located via the links provided in Table 11 and at the end of this book (see p. 146).

Adults and children over the age of 12 years (see Figure 17 and abbreviations p. vii)[35]

Step 1

Patients who present with occasional symptoms or symptoms that are only brought on by occasional exercise may be managed by inhaled short-acting β_2-agonist bronchodilators taken when necessary (prn). However, any underlying inflammation will not be treated and protector or preventer medication should be added in the case of frequent use of the relievers.

Most patients with persisting symptoms will require regular inhaled corticosteroids as the cornerstone of their treatment.

Step 2

In addition to short-acting β_2-agonist bronchodilators used on a prn basis, regular low-dose inhaled corticosteroids are added, in a dose of 200–800 mcg daily BDP/BUD equivalent. FP and the CFC-free version of BDP are considered equipotent to these at half the microgram dose. MF dosage is equipotent to FP and twice as potent as BUD and BDP, based on changes in FEV_1 from baseline.[61-63]

Step 3

Where control is still inadequate and inhaler technique and compliance have been confirmed, a regular long-acting β_2-agonist bronchodilator (salmeterol or formoterol) should be added to the low-dose steroid.

Following this measure, the control of asthma should be reassessed after about 6 weeks. If control is good, the long-acting β_2-agonist bronchodilator should be continued. If there is benefit from the addition of the long-acting β_2-agonist but control is still inadequate, the low-dose inhaled corticosteroid should be increased to the maximum recommended at step 2 (800 mcg daily BDP/BUD equivalent).

If there is no benefit from the addition of the long-acting β_2-agonist, it should be stopped and the inhaled corticosteroid should be increased to a maximum of 800 mcg/day (BDP/BUD equivalent). If control is still poor, there should be a trial of a leukotriene receptor antagonist or a sustained release theophylline. Some guidelines advocate the use of anticholinergic preparations in this step, as add-on therapy.[49]

The great majority of people with asthma will fall into the step 2 and 3 categories.

Step 4

At this stage the patient would be considered to have severe asthma. Trials should be instituted of an increased dose of inhaled corticosteroid to a maximum of 2000 mcg/day (BDP/BUD equivalent), or the addition of another therapy such as a leukotriene receptor antagonist, sustained release theophylline or a β_2-agonist tablet. Some guidelines advocate the use of anticholinergic preparations in this step, as add-on therapy.[49]

Step 5

At this stage a patient may need a regular daily dose of an oral corticosteroid, titrated to the lowest dose to control the disease as much as possible. High-dose inhaled corticosteroids should be continued and other treatments to reduce steroid use should be considered. At steps 4 and 5, patients should be referred to a specialist in the care of asthma.

Children aged 5–12 years

Step 1

Children who present with occasional symptoms or symptoms that are only brought on by occasional exercise may be managed by inhaled short-acting β_2-agonist bronchodilators taken when necessary (prn). However, any underlying inflammation will not be treated and protector or preventer medication should be added in the case of frequent use of the relievers.

Most patients with persisting symptoms will require regular inhaled corticosteroids as the cornerstone of their treatment.

Step 2

In addition to short-acting β_2-agonists used on a prn basis, regular low-dose inhaled corticosteroids are added, in a dose of 200–400 mcg daily (BDP/BUD equivalent). Guidelines advise health professionals to initiate therapy at the dose of inhaled corticosteroid considered appropriate for the control of the asthma.

Step 3

Where control is still inadequate, a regular long-acting β_2-agonist (salmeterol or formoterol) should be added to the low-dose steroid. The step 3 guidelines for children aged 5–12 years follow the same drug pathway as for adults, except for the fact that the maximum recommended dose of inhaled corticosteroid is 400 mcg/day (BDP/BUD equivalent).

The great majority of children will fall into the step 2 and 3 categories.

Step 4

Increase the dose of inhaled corticosteroid to a maximum of 800 mcg/day (BDP/BUD equivalent). These children should ideally be referred for a second opinion from a specialist in the care of paediatric asthma.

Step 5

These children may need a regular daily dose of an oral corticosteroid, titrated to the lowest dose to control the disease as much as possible. Inhaled corticosteroids should be continued at a level of 800 mcg/day (BDP/BUD equivalent).

These children should ideally be referred for a second opinion from a specialist in the care of paediatric asthma.

Children less than 5 years

Stepwise management follows the same principles as for older children. At step 2 the maximum daily dose of inhaled corticosteroid is 400 mcg/day and, in these children, leukotriene receptor antagonists are advised if inhaled steroid cannot be used (see Figure 19).

Stepping down therapy

At all steps, for all age groups, asthma control should be reviewed regularly so that treatment may be titrated appropriately. Patients whose asthma is well controlled for a period of 3 months should be considered for reduction of their therapy (removal of drugs or reduction of dose by approximately 25% each time).

Management of exacerbations

Although recommended in previous guidelines for both adults and children, review of the evidence in the UK guidelines[35] has failed to provide any support for the practice of doubling the dose of inhaled corticosteroids at the onset of an exacerbation. However, there are not many studies in this field and therefore the available evidence may not reflect the benefits of increasing the dose of inhaled steroids during exacerbations. Other experts in this field do, however, recommend and justify the practice of increasing the dose of inhaled steroids during exacerbations.[64] Many clinicians have subjective evidence of benefit derived by patients through increasing inhaled steroid medication during exacerbations. The BTS/SIGN guidelines recommend increased use of reliever β_2-agonist bronchodilator, and if this is inadequate or the exacerbation is severe, adding a short course of oral corticosteroids. All patients deteriorating during acute exacerbations should be considered for referral to a secondary care centre for treatment and monitoring. In addition, all patients treated for asthma exacerbations should be monitored frequently, to determine the effectiveness of the medication, ideally assisted by symptom and PEF diary charts.[65,66]

Table 12. Management of acute asthma in the pre-hospital setting
Primary care setting
Presentation
Management • Acute • Referral
Follow-up

Acute management of asthma

Prevention is always better than cure. Many asthma attacks can be prevented through adequate education to ensure early recognition of symptoms of poor asthma control (see Table 12). Essentially, there are three educational messages that patients need to understand in order to prevent the development of attacks. These are:

- that symptoms should respond quickly to short-acting reliever bronchodilators;
- the effects of these drugs should last at least 4 hours; and
- that changes in peak flow of over 20% compared to the best or usual reading are also indicative of poor asthma control.

Any of these three circumstances, particularly if combined with disturbed sleep due to asthma, indicate that there is a need for urgent medical advice and for the patient to implement a predetermined self-management (or action) plan.

The overall principles of management of acute or uncontrolled asthma are:[35]

- assess and act promptly in acute asthma;
- admit patients with any feature of a life-threatening or near fatal attack, or severe attack persisting after initial treatment;
- measure oxygen saturation;

- use of steroid tablets should be considered in all cases of acute asthma;
- primary care follow-up is required promptly after acute asthma.

Primary care setting

Many patients are seen in appointments lasting 8–10 minutes and, in this time, a diagnosis needs to be made, treatment needs to be initiated and decisions need to be taken on the need for referral for further investigations and treatment if necessary. Therefore, a systematic approach may be very helpful, or some would even say absolutely essential, to enable a rapid assessment and initiation of treatment, particularly in the case of acute asthma (see Table 13).

Consultation numbers for asthma episodes seem to be declining according to weekly data (Figure 21) collected by the Royal College of General Practice (RCGP) Research Department in Birmingham, UK.[67] These data do not seem to indicate a shift in diagnosis from asthma to bronchitis and it is unclear why fewer people seem to be consulting UK GPs for uncontrolled asthma. We are unaware of similar data from other countries and assume the reasons for this phenomenon are possibly related to the high rate of prescription of inhaled steroids in the UK. Of note, worldwide asthma prevalence data (see Figures 2–4) reveals a higher death rate from asthma where the prevalence has

Table 13. Process of assessment and management of acute asthma in primary care
Diagnose acute/uncontrolled asthma
Assess severity
Initiate treatment
Monitor progress
Decide on outcome (home or hospital admission)
Arrange follow-up

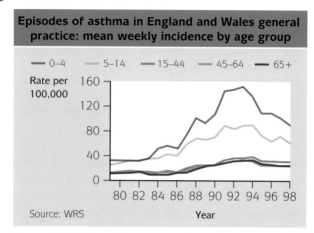

Figure 21. RCGP weekly returns – asthma episodes.
Reproduced with permission from the Lung and Asthma
Information Agency. Factsheet 2000/1, Acute Bronchitis.
www.laia.ac.uk (last accessed February 2004).

been identified as low by the relatively low prescription
rates for inhaled steroids. It is clear that, although asthma
deaths are declining in the UK and management of
asthma has improved, acute asthma is still not ideally
managed according to national guidelines. A confidential
enquiry[3,35] into the circumstances of 95 asthma deaths
found that routine clinical management was appropriate
in 59% and management of the final attack satisfactory
in 71% of these patients. While these data indicate
improvements compared to a previous confidential
enquiry, a significant proportion of the patients were not
managed appropriately. The authors of this study
advocated greater use of PEF recordings (particularly
during acute attacks, to document recovery), prescription
monitoring of the underuse of inhaled corticosteroids,
consideration of the use of combined preparations where
persistent overuse of bronchodilators is occurring, and
increased input for young patients whose routine
management is proving difficult.

Mode of presentation

Any patient with known asthma, consulting for respiratory symptoms, may in fact be developing an acute asthma exacerbation. While diagnosis is usually straightforward where patients present with typical features of uncontrolled asthma, such as wheezing, cough and difficulty breathing, sometimes the presentation can be less clear. Furthermore, many patients do not present with typical features, and sometimes patients at risk of dying from their attack do not demonstrate any of the usual danger signs.[35]

Receptionists working in primary care are often the first point of contact for patients with a history of asthma, who present with respiratory symptoms or saying their asthma is out of control. These people need to be dealt with sympathetically and booked in to see the doctor or asthma nurse urgently. In order for patients to be seen urgently and appropriately, the receptionists need adequate training in addition to the patients themselves, whose action plan should include details that they should explain clearly when booking an appointment, that their asthma is out of control and they need urgent attention.

Once patients see the physician or asthma nurse, the diagnosis needs to be confirmed. In contrast with the secondary care setting, patients presenting in primary care do not arrive with a referral letter, indicating the nature of the problem. Patients presenting for the first time with an asthma attack, before their asthma has been diagnosed, pose particular problems for doctors and nurses working in primary care. It is often difficult to differentiate cardiac from respiratory causes of breathlessness, and to decide whether the cause of the problem is an infection rather than acute asthma. Often the diagnosis is unclear, and treatment needs to be symptomatic with a clear diagnosis to follow later, either in primary or secondary care.

In patients previously diagnosed with asthma, suspicion of poor asthma control is aroused by the presence of respiratory symptoms, particularly at night or during exercise, with or without a history of poor response to the

Table 14. Initial assessments – the role of symptoms, signs and measurements	
Clinical features	Clinical features, symptoms and respiratory and cardiovascular signs helpful in recognizing severe asthma, but none specific, and their absence does not exclude a severe attack
PEF or FEV$_1$	Measurements of airway calibre improve recognition of severity and guide hospital or home management decisions. PEF is more convenient and cheaper than FEV$_1$. PEF as % previous best value or % predicted most useful
Pulse oximetry	Necessary to determine adequacy of oxygen therapy and need for arterial blood gas measurement. Aim of oxygen therapy is to maintain SpO$_2$ ≥ 92%
Blood gases (ABG)	Necessary for patients with SpO$_2$ < 92% or other features of life-threatening asthma
Chest X-ray	Not routinely recommended in patients in the absence of: • Suspected pneumomediastinum or pneumothorax • Suspected consolidation • Life-threatening asthma • Failure to respond to treatment satisfactorily • Requirement for ventilation
Systolic paradox	Abandoned as an indicator of the severity of an attack

Source (Tables 14 and 15): British Thoracic Society/SIGN (www. brit-thoracic.org.uk/sign/index.htm). Reproduced from: British guidelines on the management of asthma. *Thorax* 2003; **58**(Suppl 1): i1–i94.[35]

usual medication. Patients with an asthma action plan, who present with a peak flow diary chart, may provide additional assistance for the physician making the diagnosis.

Table 15. Levels of severity of acute asthma exacerbations in adults

Near fatal asthma	Raised P_aCO_2 and/or requiring mechanical ventilation with raised inflation pressures
Life-threatening asthma	Any one of the following in a patient with severe asthma: • PEF < 33% best or predicted • SpO_2 < 92% • P_aO_2 < 8 kPa • Normal P_aCO_2 (4.6–6.0 kPa) • Silent chest • Cyanosis • Feeble respiratory effort • Bradycardia • Dysrhythmia • Hypotension • Exhaustion • Confusion • Coma
Acute severe asthma	Any one of: • PEF 33–50% best or predicted • Respiratory rate ≥ 25/min • Heart rate ≥ 110/min • Inability to complete sentences in one breath
Moderate asthma exacerbation	• Increasing symptoms • PEF > 50–75% best or predicted • No features of acute severe asthma
Brittle asthma	• Type 1: wide PEF variability (> 40% diurnal variation for >50% of the time over a period > 150 days) despite intensive therapy • Type 2: sudden severe attacks on a background of apparently well-controlled asthma

Table 16. Initial assessment of acute asthma in children aged > 2 years in general practice

Moderate exacerbation	Severe exacerbation	Life-threatening exacerbation
• $SpO_2 \geq 92\%$	• $SpO_2 < 92\%$	• $SpO_2 < 92\%$
• PEF $\geq$ 50% best/predicted (> 5 years)	• PEF $\geq$ 50% best/predicted (> 5 years)	• PEF $\geq$ 50% best/predicted (> 5 years)
• Able to talk	• Too breathless to talk	• Silent chest
• Heart rate: – $\leq$ 130/min (2–5 years) – $\leq$ 120/min (> 5 years)	• Heart rate: – > 130/min (2–5 years) – > 120/min (> 5 years)	• Poor respiratory effort
Respiratory rate: – $\leq$ 50/min (2–5 years) – $\leq$ 30/min (> 5 years)	• Respiratory rate: – > 50/min (2–5 years) – > 30/min (> 5 years)	• Agitation
		• Altered consciousness
	• Use of accessory neck muscles	• Cyanosis

Measure PEF or FEV_1 in all children aged > 5 years

Source: British Thoracic Society/SIGN (www.brit-thoracic.org.uk/sign/index.htm). Reproduced from: British guidelines on the management of asthma. *Thorax* 2003; **58**(Suppl 1): i1–i94.[35]

Assessment (see Table 14)[35] should include the patient's level of distress (difficulty breathing, difficulty in speaking, exhaustion and level of consciousness), clinical examination (pulse, respirations, use of accessory respiratory muscles, presence of cyanosis), auscultation of the lungs and lung function (peak expiratory flow or spirometry), and pulse oximetry (see Tables 15 and 16)[35] can then be used to grade the severity of the attack and facilitate the treatment necessary. The clinician should, however, be aware that some patients with acute, life-threatening attacks of asthma may

Table 17. Patients at risk of developing near fatal or fatal asthma

A combination of severe asthma:

Recognized by one or more of:	and	Adverse behavioural or psychosocial features
• Previous near fatal asthma (previous ventilation or respiratory acidosis)		• Non-compliance with treatment or monitoring
		• Failure to attend appointments
• Previous asthma admission		• Self-discharge from hospital
• Requiring ≥ 3 classes of asthma medication		• Psychosis, depression, other psychiatric illness or deliberate self-harm
• Heavy use of β_2-agonist		• Current or recent major tranquillizer use
• Repeated attendances at A&E for asthma care		• Denial
		• Alcohol or drug abuse
• Brittle asthma		• Obesity
		• Learning difficulties
		• Employment problems
		• Income problems
		• Social isolation
		• Childhood abuse
		• Severe domestic, marital or legal stress

Source: British Thoracic Society/SIGN (www.brit-thoracic.org.uk/sign/index.htm). Reproduced from: British guidelines on the management of asthma. *Thorax* 2003; **58**(Suppl 1): i1–i94.[35]

not demonstrate any of the features listed in Table 17.[35] Therefore, any patient with a history of asthma, consulting for respiratory symptoms, should be taken very seriously.

Table 18. Who should be admitted to hospital with acute asthma?[3,35]

Admit to hospital if any:

- life-threatening features
- features of acute severe asthma present after initial treatment
- previous near fatal asthma

Lower threshold for admission if:

- afternoon or evening attack
- recent nocturnal symptoms or hospital admission
- previous severe attacks
- patient unable to assess progress of own condition (identify deterioration)
- concern over social circumstances

Table 19. Immediate treatment of acute asthma[35]

High doses of short-acting β_2-agonists

- Ideally via oxygen-driven nebulizer (salbutamol: adults, 5 mg; 2–5 years, 2.5 mg; > 5 years, 5 mg; terbutaline: adults, 10 mg; 2–5 years, 5 mg; > 5 years, 10 mg)
- Or via spacer/air-driven nebulizer (1 puff 10–20 times)

Oxygen (40–60%)

Steroids

- Oral prednisolone: adults, 50 mg; 2–5 years, 20 mg; > 5 years, 30–40 mg

Treatment of acute asthma

Once the diagnosis has been made, two decisions need to be taken: (i) What treatment is needed? (ii) Does the patient need to go to hospital? (See Tables 18 and 19.) This latter question is important because, in order to save time, an ambulance needs to be called immediately if the severity of the attack warrants this. Another factor in primary care is that there will often be many other patients waiting to be attended to and the sooner the person with acute asthma is sent safely off to hospital, the sooner these others can be attended to.

The BTS/SIGN guidelines provide detailed evidence-based recommendations for the management of each level of severity of acute asthma in adults and children. These are shown in Tables 20–22.

Table 20. Management of acute asthma in children aged over 2 years in general practice		
Moderate exacerbation	**Severe exacerbation**	**Life-threatening exacerbation**
• β_2-Agonist 2–4 puffs via spacer ± facemask	• Oxygen via facemask	• Oxygen via facemask

• Consider soluble prednisolone:
  – 20 mg (2–5 years)
  – 30–40 mg (> 5 years)
	• β_2-Agonist 2–4 puffs via spacer ± facemask or nebulized salbutamol (2–5 years: 2.5 mg; > 5 years: 5 mg) or terbutaline (2–5 years: 5 mg; > 5 years: 10 mg)	• Nebulized salbutamol (2–5 years: 2.5 mg; > 5 years: 5 mg) or terbutaline (2–5 years: 5 mg; > 5 years: 10 mg)

Increase β_2-agonist dose by 2 puffs every 2 minutes up to 10 puffs according to response	• Soluble prednisolone:
	  – 20 mg (2–5 years)
	  – 30–40 mg (> 5 years)
		• Ipratropium (0.25 mg)
		
		• Soluble prednisolone (2–5 years: 20 mg; > 5 years: 30–40 mg) or i.v. hydrocortisone (2–5 years: 50 mg; > 5 years: 100 mg)

	Assess response to treatment 15 minutes after β_2-agonist	

Source: British Thoracic Society/SIGN (www.brit-thoracic.org.uk/sign/index.htm). Reproduced from: British guidelines on the management of asthma. *Thorax* 2003; **58**(Suppl 1): i1–i94.[35]

Table 21. Assessment and management of acute asthma in adults in general practice

Moderate asthma	Acute severe asthma	Life-threatening asthma
Initial assessment		
PEF > 50% best or predicted	PEF 33–50% best or predicted	PEF < 33% best or predicted
Further assessment		
• Speech normal	• Cannot complete sentences	• SpO_2 < 92%
• Respiration < 25 breaths/min	• Respiration ≥ 25 breaths/min	• Silent chest, cyanosis or poor respiratory effort
• Pulse < 110 beats/min	• Pulse ≥ 110 beats/min	• Bradycardia, dysrhythmia or hypotension
		• Exhaustion, confusion or coma
Management		
Treat at home or in surgery and ASSESS RESPONSE TO TREATMENT	Consider admission	Arrange immediate ADMISSION

Source: British Thoracic Society/SIGN (www.brit-thoracic.org.uk/sign/index.htm). Reproduced from: British guidelines on the management of asthma. *Thorax* 2003; **58**(Suppl 1): i1–i94.[35]

A chart (see Figure 22)[36,68] may be helpful in assessing and treating a patient in primary care. This could then be photocopied and sent with the patient in the event that hospital admission is required. This is particularly helpful in the case of young children, who may appear much better after initial treatment once they arrive in the emergency department. Many children are discharged home too early in these circumstances.

Table 22. Steroids and other therapy for acute asthma in adults

Give steroid tablets in adequate doses in all cases of acute asthma

Continue prednisolone (40–50 mg daily) for at least 5 days or until recovery

Nebulized ipratropium bromide (0.5 mg, 4–6 hourly) should be added to β_2-agonist treatment if poor response to β_2-agonist therapy

Consider i.v. magnesium sulphate for patients with poorly responding acute severe or life-threatening asthma

I.v. magnesium sulphate (1.2–2 g i.v. infusion over 20 minutes) and i.v. aminophylline should only be used following consultation with senior medical staff

Routine prescription of antibiotics is not indicated for acute asthma

Source: British Thoracic Society/SIGN (www.brit-thoracic.org.uk/ sign/index.htm). Reproduced from: British guidelines on the management of asthma. *Thorax* 2003; **58**(Suppl 1): i1–i94.[35]

Follow-up

It is a mistake to assume, as many do, that the acute management is the most important aspect of care for patients suffering from exacerbations. It is just as important to ensure that adequate follow-up occurs. Patients should be followed up, preferably within primary care, until the episode has resolved. Therefore, a system needs to be in place that ensures the primary health care team are well informed when patients are seen in the Accident and Emergency Hospital Departments or due for hospital discharge.

It is often difficult for the health professional as well as the patient to decide when an acute attack or exacerbation of asthma has resolved. Peak flow diaries may be very helpful, both in determining when it is safe to reduce or stop oral steroids and also in educating patients of the value of these measurements. During the recovery phase of an attack, the readings may fluctuate, thus illustrating some of the danger signs for patients.

A flow chart for managing asthma exacerbations in primary care

This chart could be photocopied and included with a referral letter when admitting children to hospital (This chart is intended for monitoring patients in the pre-hospital setting, to act as an aide-mémoire as well as supplementary documentation for referral to hospital)

Name: ....

Date: .... / .... / ....

DOB: .... / .... / ....   Best previous PEF: ....

Time first seen: ____ H ____

History: ....

Time	Pulse rate	Resp. rate	Using accessory muscles (children)	PEF	Pulse oximetry (SpO₂)	Cyanosis	Exhaustion	Oxygen flow rate	Treatment
___ H ___			SCM y/n Scalini y/n Alae nasi y/n Intercostals y/n			Y/N		___ l/M	Salbutamol/Terbutaline/Atrovent Dose: **Delivery:** Nebulizer/Spacer Oral Steroid: ____ Inhaled steroid: ____
___ H ___			SCM y/n Scalini y/n Alae nas y/n Intercostals y/n			Y/N		___ l/M	Salbutamol/Terbutaline/Atrovent Dose: **Delivery:** Nebulizer/Spacer Oral Steroid: ____ Inhaled steroid: ____
___ H ___			SCM y/n Scalini y/n Alae nasi y/n Intercostals y/n			Y/N		___ l/M	Salbutamol/Terbutaline/Atrovent Dose: **Delivery:** Nebulizer/Spacer Oral Steroid: ____ Inhaled steroid: ____
___ H ___			SCM y/n Scalini y/n Alae nasi y/n Intercostals y/n			Y/N		___ l/M	Salbutamol/Terbutaline/Atrovent Dose: **Delivery:** Nebulizer/Spacer Oral Steroid: ____ Inhaled steroid: ____

SCM = Sternocleidomastoid muscles

Figure 22. Primary care acute asthma assessment. © Levy M, Hilton S. *Asthma in Practice*, 4th edn. London: Royal College of General Practitioners, 2000.[36]

Delivery devices

Inhaler devices

For many years inhalation has been the preferred mode of administration of drugs for asthma, because this route offers several advantages. The drug is delivered directly to the affected organ, without undergoing systemic absorption, thus permitting a lower dose of medication to be used, reducing the potential for adverse side-effects.

The common feature of all inhalation devices is that they are designed to deliver the medication in particles of respirable size – that is, of a size appropriate for delivery to the medium and small airways. This is generally agreed to be less than 5 µm. Particles larger than this may have difficulty in entering the small airways. A number of factors influence successful drug delivery[69] (see Table 23).

The most common reasons for failure of inhaled drugs are inappropriate device selection, incorrect inhaler technique or lack of compliance. Even people who use a device well may forget how to use it, or be unable to use it when in a stressful situation such as an asthma attack. People are expected to absorb a lot of information when seeing a health professional; a stepwise approach during

Table 23. Inhaler devices
Inhaler design variables
Different formulations of drugs
Mechanical activation
Internal resistance to airflow
Patient variables
Pulmonary performance (exacerbation of disease vs normality)
Ability to learn/be taught correct technique
Physical size of lungs (child vs adult)
Effort varies from dose to dose

Table 24. A stepwise approach to teaching patients about inhaler devices
Discussion of disease and management
Counselling where appropriate
Device selection
Demonstration of correct usage
Supervised device handling
Check correct inspiratory flow rate for selected device
Supervised reading of patient instruction leaflet
Instructions regarding storage and cleaning
Joint agreement between health professional and patient on self-management programme
Check patient's understanding, compliance and inhaler technique at subsequent consultations

the consultation may assist in improving mutual understanding (Table 24).

At present, there are three main methods of delivering inhaled medications: these include pressurized metered dose inhalers (pMDIs), dry powder inhalers (DPIs) and nebulizers.

Pressurized metered dose inhalers
Pressurized metered dose inhalers (pMDIs) consist of a plastic container within which is a pressurized canister containing the medication (see Figure 23). When the canister is pressed (or actuated) a metered dose of the drug is released in aerosol form. Actuation may be manual or automatic as the patient inspires, depending on the device. If the canister is actuated manually the patient must inhale while the drug is being released. This requires a degree of coordination, which many patients find difficult and which will be beyond the ability of others (e.g. some children or elderly people). The inspiration must also be slow and at a low inspiratory flow rate (20–40 litres/minute), otherwise most of the respirable dose will be lost by impaction on the

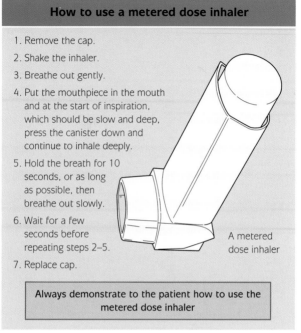

How to use a metered dose inhaler

1. Remove the cap.
2. Shake the inhaler.
3. Breathe out gently.
4. Put the mouthpiece in the mouth and at the start of inspiration, which should be slow and deep, press the canister down and continue to inhale deeply.
5. Hold the breath for 10 seconds, or as long as possible, then breathe out slowly.
6. Wait for a few seconds before repeating steps 2–5.
7. Replace cap.

A metered dose inhaler

Always demonstrate to the patient how to use the metered dose inhaler

Figure 23. Metered dose inhaler (pMDI). Reproduced with kind permission by the National Respiratory Training Centre, Warwick, UK (www.nrtc.org.uk).

back of the throat. Very careful instruction is therefore needed if they are to be used optimally, as studies show[70,71] that both health professionals and patients find difficulty in using pMDIs optimally. However, their small size and portability makes them popular with patients.

In an attempt to assist patients who struggle with coordinating the use of a pMDI, a chamber device (small or large volume) may be used. There are a range of spacer devices available, produced by different manufacturers, not all compatible with each other (see Figures 24–26). Following the actuation of the canister the medication remains in suspension in the chamber for a short time, allowing the patient to inhale the drug by tidal breathing.

How to use a spacer device e.g. Nebuhaler

Method particularly useful for young children

1. Remove the cap, shake the inhaler and insert into the device.

2. Place the mouthpiece in the child's mouth (if using the Nebuhaler be careful the the child's lips are behind the ring).

3. Seal the child's lips round the mouthpiece by gently placing the fingers of one hand round the lips.

4. Encourage the child to breathe in and out slowly and gently (this will make a "clicking" sound as the valve opens and closes).

5. Once the breathing pattern is well established, depress the canister with the free hand and leave the device in the same position as the child continues to breathe several more times. The child should take five breaths for each puff of medication.

6. Remove the device from the child's mouth.

7. For a second dose wait a few seconds and repeat steps 1–6.

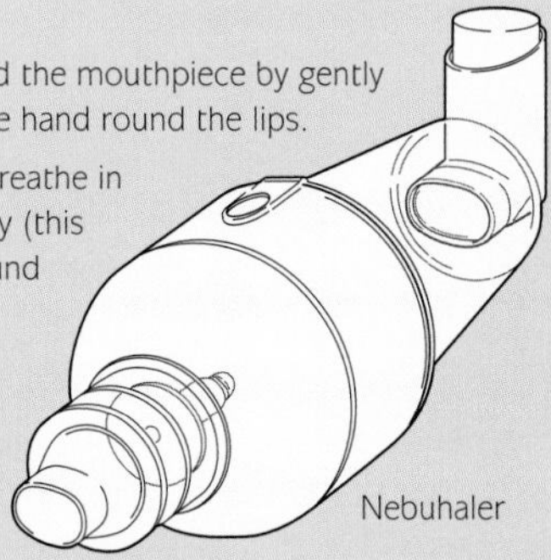

Nebuhaler

Always demonstrate to the patient how to use the Nebuhaler

Figure 24. Large volume spacer – Nebuhaler. Reproduced with kind permission by the National Respiratory Training Centre, Warwick, UK (www.nrtc.org.uk).

The dose should be inhaled within 10 seconds, as settling of the drug reduces deposition. Single rather than multiple actuations should be used, as the latter will reduce the drug available for inhalation.[72] Retention of the larger particles in the device reduces systemic deposition. Although these devices are more effective and easier to use than metered dose inhalers alone, they are bulky and may have restrictions in terms of acceptability and lifestyle. The plastic spacers should be washed and air-dried, as static can reduce the

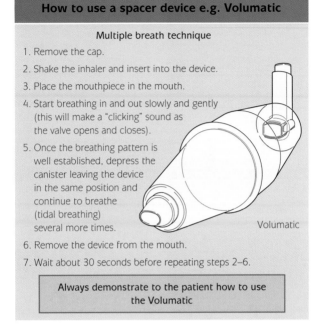

How to use a spacer device e.g. Volumatic

Multiple breath technique

1. Remove the cap.
2. Shake the inhaler and insert into the device.
3. Place the mouthpiece in the mouth.
4. Start breathing in and out slowly and gently (this will make a "clicking" sound as the valve opens and closes).
5. Once the breathing pattern is well established, depress the canister leaving the device in the same position and continue to breathe (tidal breathing) several more times.

Volumatic

6. Remove the device from the mouth.
7. Wait about 30 seconds before repeating steps 2–6.

> Always demonstrate to the patient how to use the Volumatic

Figure 25. Large volume spacer – Volumatic. Reproduced with kind permission by the National Respiratory Training Centre, Warwick, UK (www.nrtc.org.uk).

available drug by half.[73] Spacers are important in the treatment of acute severe asthma; they are as effective as a nebulizer for administering β_2-agonist medication.

For children too small to close their mouths around the mouthpiece of the chamber device, a mask may be added (see Figure 27). The mask is closely applied to the infant's face, as a gap greater than 1 cm between mask and face will result in a greatly diminished drug deposition. The infant then inhales the drug by tidal breathing.

How to use the Aerochamber

Method for patient who can use the device without help

1. Remove the cap.

2. Shake the inhaler and insert in the back of the Aerochamber.

3. Place the mouthpiece in the mouth (or the mask over mouth and nose).

4. Press the canister once to release a dose of the drug.

5. Take a deep, slow breath in (if you hear a whistling sound, you are breathing in too quickly).

6. Hold the breath for about 10 seconds, then breathe out through the mouthpiece.

7. Breathe in again but do not press the canister.

8. Remove the mouthpiece from the mouth and breathe out.

9. Wait a few seconds before a second dose is taken, and repeat steps 2–8.

Method particularly useful for young children

1. Remove the cap.

2. Shake the inhaler and insert in the back of the Aerochamber.

3. Place the mouthpiece in the mouth (or the mask over mouth and nose).

4. Encourage the child to gently breathe in (if you hear a whistling sound, the child is breathing in too quickly*).

Aerochamber

5. Once the breathing pattern is well established, depress the canister with the free hand and leave the canister in the same position as the child continues to breathe in and out slowly five more times.

6. Remove the Aerochamber from the child's mouth.

7. For a second dose, wait a few seconds and repeat steps 2–6.

*NB. The child Aerochamber device with mask and infant Aerochamber device do not whistle.

> **Always demonstrate to the patient how to use the Aerochamber**

Figure 26. Large volume spacer – Aerochamber. Reproduced with kind permission by the National Respiratory Training Centre, Warwick, UK (www.nrtc.org.uk).

How to use the Nebuchamber

1. Remove the protective cap from the aerosol inhaler.
2. Shake the inhaler so the contents are well mixed.
3. Place the mouthpiece of the aerosol inhaler into the small oval opening of the spacer.
4. Keeping the spacer level, place the mouthpiece between your teeth and close your lips around it.
5. Press (activate) the inhaler canister once and breathe in slowly and deeply through your mouth.
6. For each additional dose of inhaler medication, remove the inhaler from the spacer and repeat steps 2–5.
7. Remove the inhaler from the spacer and replace the protective inhaler cap.
8. Replace spacer in storage bag.

NB. It may be preferable and easier for the younger age group child to take five breaths in and out (tidal breathing) to each actuation. The elderly may find it easier too.

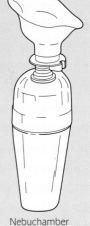

Nebuchamber

Always demonstrate to the patient how to use the Nebuchamber

Figure 27. Large volume spacer with mask – Nebuchamber. Reproduced with kind permission by the National Respiratory Training Centre, Warwick, UK (www.nrtc.org.uk).

How to use the Easi-breathe

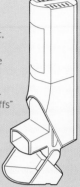

1. Shake the inhaler.
2. Hold the inhaler upright. Open the cap.
3. Breathe out gently. Keep the inhaler upright, put the mouthpiece in the mouth and close lips and teeth around it (the air holes on the top must not be blocked by the hand).
4. Breathe in steadily through the mouthpiece. DON'T stop breathing when the inhaler "puffs" and continue taking a really deep breath.
5. Hold the breath for about 10 seconds.
6. After use, hold the inhaler upright and immediately close the cap.
7. For a second dose, wait a few seconds before repeating steps 1–6.

Easi-breathe

Always demonstrate to the patient how to use the Easi-breathe

Figure 28. Breath-actuated pMDI. Reproduced with kind permission by the National Respiratory Training Centre, Warwick, UK (www.nrtc.org.uk).

A further variant of the pMDI is the patient-actuated device (see Figure 28) and Autohaler™, not shown. It uses energy from the aerosol to disperse medication; the aerosol release is triggered at a predetermined inspiratory flow rate and drug delivery is dependent on the ability to achieve the trigger flow rate. It is important that the person continues to inspire when the flow rate is triggered.

These devices have an advantage over the conventional press and breathe pMDIs, as they take away the need to coordinate actuation and inspiration, and may be suitable for patients who have difficulty in this.

Dry powder inhalers

Dry powder inhalers (DPIs) contain the medication in powder form, either in a reservoir or in sealed blisters. The patient's inhalation activates these devices, and they are

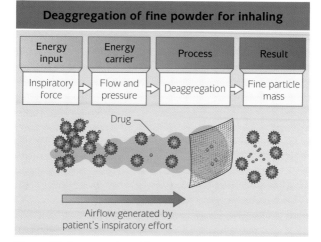

Deaggregation of fine powder for inhaling

Energy input	Energy carrier	Process	Result
Inspiratory force	Flow and pressure	Deaggregation	Fine particle mass

Drug

Airflow generated by patient's inspiratory effort

Figure 29. Deaggregation of fine powder for inhaling. Reproduced from Chrystyn H. Is inhalation rate important for a dry powder inhaler? Using the In-Check Dial to identify these rates. *Respir Med* 2003; **97**(2): 181–187 with permission from Elsevier Limited.

known as patient-activated devices. The patient's inhalation draws the medication from the delivery chamber and into the lungs. Unlike the pMDIs, where the device itself produces the aerosolized drug, with the dry powder inhalers it is the force of the inhalation or inspiratory flow rate that deaggregates the powder into particles of respirable size. The force needed to produce this effect varies according to the design of the device. Some dry powder inhalers will have a higher internal resistance than others in order to deaggregate the particular drug in the particular device (see Figure 29).

As the dry powder devices are patient activated, there is no need for coordinating activation and inhalation. However, careful instruction is needed to ensure that the patient primes the device and can achieve the optimal inspiratory flow rate for the particular device. Dry powder devices are suitable for a wide range of patients, but are generally unsuitable for children under the age of 5, as their inspiratory flow rate is likely to be variable. They are generally small and portable (see Figures 30–37).

How to use the Accuhaler

1. Open the Accuhaler by holding its outer casing in one hand whilst pushing the thumbgrip away until a click is heard.

2. Hold the Accuhaler with the mouthpiece towards you and slide the lever away until it clicks. This makes the dose available for inhalation and moves the dose counter on.

3. Holding the Accuhaler level, breathe out gently away from the device, put mouthpiece in mouth and take a breath in steadily and deeply.

4. Remove the Accuhaler from mouth and hold breath for about 10 seconds.

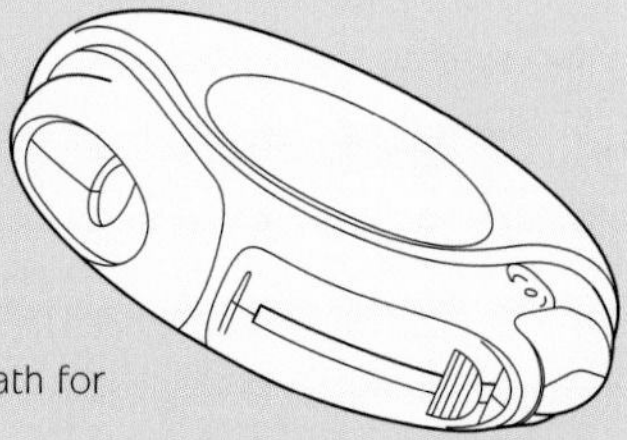

Accuhaler

5. To close, slide the thumbgrip back towards you as far as it will go until it clicks.

6. For a second dose, repeat steps 1–5.

7. The dose counter counts down from 60 to 0. The last five numbers are red.

Always demonstrate to the patient how to use the Accuhaler

Figure 30. Dry powder inhaler – Accuhaler™. Reproduced with kind permission by the National Respiratory Training Centre, Warwick, UK (www.nrtc.org.uk).

How to use the Turbohaler

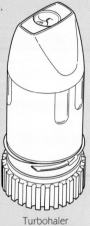

1. Unscrew and lift off white cover.

2. Hold Turbohaler upright and twist the grip, then twist it back again as far as it will go. You should hear a click.

3. Breathe out gently, put the mouthpiece between the lips and teeth and breathe in as deeply as possible. Even when a full dose is taken there may be no taste (do not breathe out into Turbohaler).

4 Remove the Turbohaler from the mouth and hold breath for about 10 seconds.

5. For a second dose, repeat steps 2–4.

6. Replace white cover.

7. A red line appears in the window on the side of the Turbohaler when there are 20 doses left. When the whole window is red the inhaler is empty.

Turbohaler

Always demonstrate to the patient how to use the Turbohaler

Figure 31. Dry powder inhaler – Turbohaler™. Reproduced with kind permission by the National Respiratory Training Centre, Warwick, UK (www.nrtc.org.uk).

How to use the Turbohaler for combination therapy

1. Unscrew and lift off white cover.

2. Hold main body of Turbohaler upright. Twist the red base as far as it will go in both directions. A clicking sound will be heard.

3. Breathe out away from the Turbohaler mouthpiece.

4. Put the mouthpiece between the lips and teeth and breathe in as deeply as possible.

5. Remove the Turbohaler from the mouth and hold the breath for about 10 seconds or as long as is comfortable.

6. For further doses, repeat steps 2–5.

7. Replace white cover.

8. The dose counter changes from a white background to a red one once it has the number 20 in the window. When the 0 on the red background reaches the middle of the window the device is empty.

NB. Before a new device is used for the first time, prepare the inhaler as in steps 1 and 2, and repeat step 2. This is the initial priming. Thereafter, follow follow instructions 1–8.

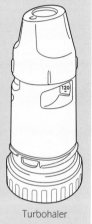

Turbohaler

> **Always demonstrate to the patient how to use the Turbohaler**

Figure 32. Dry powder inhaler – Turbohaler™ with counter. Reproduced with kind permission by the National Respiratory Training Centre, Warwick, UK (www.nrtc.org.uk).

How to use a Twisthaler

1. Before removing the cap, check counter window and pointer on cap are lined up.

2. Hold the main body of the Twisthaler, keeping it upright with the maroon base at the bottom.

3. Unscrew the white cap anticlockwise and lift off.

4. Breathe out away from the Twisthaler mouthpiece.

Twisthaler

5. Put the inhaler mouthpiece between the lips and teeth and breathe in deeply and quickly.

6. Remove the Twisthaler from the mouth and hold breath for about 10 seconds or as long as is comfortable.

7. Replace the cap after inhalation, turning it clockwise until a click is heard.

8. If other doses are required, repeat steps 1–7.

9. The amount of medication left in the device can be easily checked on the numerical counter.

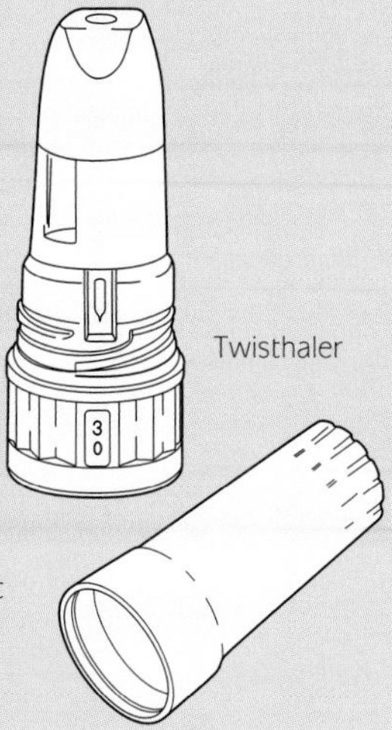

> **Always demonstrate to the patient how to use the Twisthaler**

Figure 33. Dry powder inhaler – Twisthaler™. Reproduced with kind permission by the National Respiratory Training Centre, Warwick, UK (www.nrtc.org.uk).

How to use the Diskhaler

This device takes foil-covered disks containing either four or eight measured doses

1. To load a disk, remove the mouthpiece cover, pull the white tray out by squeezing the white ridges at either side and put the disk on top with numbers uppermost.

2. Replace the tray, and rotate the disk by sliding the tray in and out until number 8 shows on the window.

3. To use the device, keeping it horizontal, lift the rear of the lid up as far as it will go, piercing the top and the bottom of the blister, then close the lid.

4. Keeping the device level, breathe out gently, close the mouth round the mouthpiece (taking care not to block the air holes at the side) and breathe in as deeply as possible.

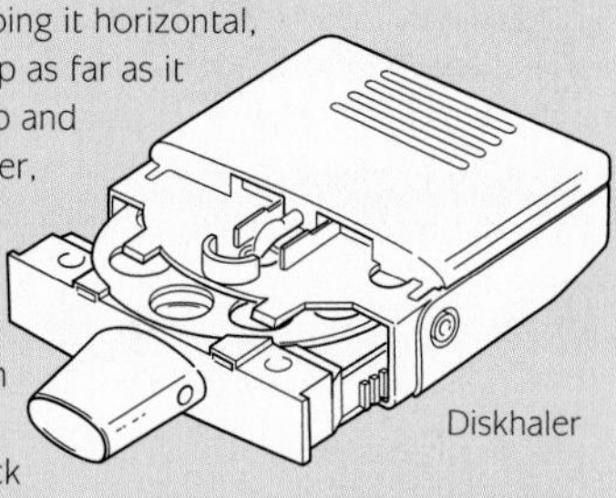

Diskhaler

5. Remove Diskhaler from the mouth and hold breath for about 10 seconds, then breathe out slowly.

6. Slide tray in and out ready for the next dose, then repeat steps 3–5.

7. Replace mouthpiece cover.

Always demonstrate to the patient how to use the Diskhaler

Figure 34. Dry powder inhaler – Diskhaler™. Reproduced with kind permission by the National Respiratory Training Centre, Warwick, UK (www.nrtc.org.uk).

How to use a Clickhaler

1. Hold the Clickhaler upright.

2. Remove the mouthpiece cover from the inhaler.

3. Shake the inhaler.

4. Continue to hold the Clickhaler upright with your thumb on the base and a finger on the coloured push button.

5. Press the dosing button down firmly (once only, then release).

6. Breathe out gently and put mouthpiece between the lips and teeth, sealing the lips around the mouthpiece (do not breathe out into the Clickhaler).

7. Breathe in steadily and deeply. Remove Clickhaler from the mouth and hold the breath for about 5–10 seconds. Breathe out slowly.

8. For a second dose, keep the Clickhaler upright and repeat steps 3–7.

9. Replace the mouthpiece cover.

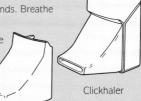

Clickhaler

10. There is a dose counter at the back of the inhaler. After 190 actuations a red warning appears in the counter window, which shows there are 10 actuations left. When no actuations are left, the inhaler locks and can no longer be used and should be discarded.

> **Always demonstrate to the patient how to use the Clickhaler**

Figure 35. Dry powder inhaler – Clickhaler™. Reproduced with kind permission by the National Respiratory Training Centre, Warwick, UK (www.nrtc.org.uk).

How to use the Aerohaler

To load

1. Open the mouthpiece by lifting it up.

2. Lift the magazine up slightly and turn it round in a clockwise direction until the mark "6" lines up with the Δ on the base. Push the magazine down again.

3. Load the capsules (either way up) into the magazine. Push down the mouthpiece until it clicks.

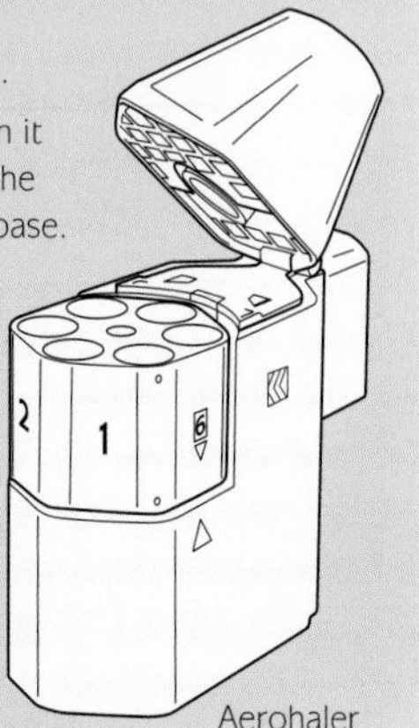

To use

1. Hold the inhaler upright. Push the white button on the side of the inhaler until it clicks and then release it immediately (this pierces the capsule).

Aerohaler

2. Breathe out gently, put the mouthpiece in the mouth and breathe in as deeply as possible.

3. Remove Aerohaler from the mouth and hold breath for about 10 seconds. Breathe out gently.

4. Turn the magazine until the next lowest number appears above the mark Δ on the base. The next dose is then ready.

5. Reload the magazine when all the capsules have been used.

> Always demonstrate to the patient how to use the Aerohaler

Figure 36. Dry powder inhaler – Aerohaler™. Reproduced with kind permission by the National Respiratory Training Centre, Warwick, UK (www.nrtc.org.uk).

Nebulizers

These devices operate by nebulizing a solution or a suspension of the drug into respirable particles. This is achieved either by forcing air through the liquid using the Venturi effect, or by ultrasonic vibration of a plate under the liquid.

How to use a Pulvinal

1. Unscrew and take off protective cover.
2. Hold Pulvinal upright.
3. Press and hold button on mouthpiece.
4. Twist base of inhaler to right, continuing to press button until red mark shows in the hole beneath the button.
5. Release the button on the mouthpiece and twist the inhaler back again in the opposite direction until it clicks and the red mark has changed to green.
6. Breathe out away from the mouthpiece, then put inhaler mouthpiece between the lips and teeth.
7. Breathe in deeply and and as quickly as possible.
8. Remove the inhaler from the mouth and hold breath for about 10 seconds.
9. If other doses are required, repeat steps 2–8.
10. The amount of medication left in the device can be easily viewed through the clear walls of the device.
11. Replace protective cover.

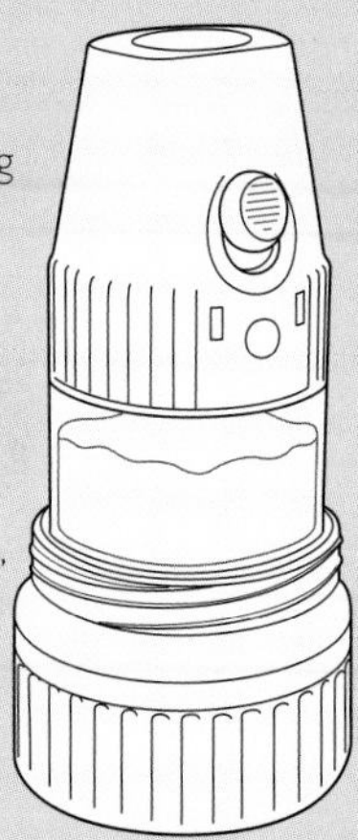

Pulvinal

Always demonstrate to the patient how to use the Pulvinal

Figure 37. Dry powder inhaler – Pulvinal™. Reproduced with kind permission by the National Respiratory Training Centre, Warwick, UK (www.nrtc.org.uk).

They are more effective at nebulizing solutions than suspensions and therefore are used more for nebulizing β_2-agonists such as salbutamol than for corticosteroids.

In asthma their use is reserved for administering large doses of β_2-agonist bronchodilators in the management of acute severe asthma. A systematic review concluded that

β_2-agonists administered by means of a pMDI and large volume chamber device (Figure 38) are as effective in the treatment of this emergency as the same dose of drug through a nebulizer;[74] therefore, if an oxygen-driven

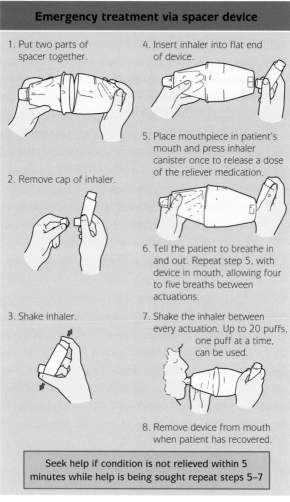

Emergency treatment via spacer device

1. Put two parts of spacer together.

2. Remove cap of inhaler.

3. Shake inhaler.

4. Insert inhaler into flat end of device.

5. Place mouthpiece in patient's mouth and press inhaler canister once to release a dose of the reliever medication.

6. Tell the patient to breathe in and out. Repeat step 5, with device in mouth, allowing four to five breaths between actuations.

7. Shake the inhaler between every actuation. Up to 20 puffs, one puff at a time, can be used.

8. Remove device from mouth when patient has recovered.

Seek help if condition is not relieved within 5 minutes while help is being sought repeat steps 5–7

Figure 38. Emergency treatment using a large volume spacer device. Reproduced with kind permission by the National Respiratory Training Centre, Warwick, UK (www.nrtc.org.uk).

nebulizer is not available, this system may be used to treat people with acute asthma.

Device selection

Device selection is of critical importance as, especially in children, incorrect or inappropriate device selection is a common reason for treatment failure.

The choice of device should be made according to the medication (or medication class) selected by the health professional, the ability of the patient to use a device effectively, and the acceptability of the device to the patient (e.g. a teenager is unlikely to wish to carry a large volume chamber device to school).

The patient should be shown the device and how to use it, with the help of the manufacturer's diagrams. The next step is to instruct and check the patient's inhalation technique. Whether a pMDI or a DPI is used, for a medication to be delivered effectively to the lungs, the patient must inhale at the appropriate time and with the appropriate inspiratory force for the particular device. It is difficult to check this aspect of device use with a placebo device, as estimations of the patient's inspiratory flow rate are likely to be inaccurate.

There are various devices available that have been developed to meet this need. The AIMS machine is used in training and assessing patients in the use of pMDIs. It measures the inspiratory flow rate, the timing of the inspiration and actuation, and the breath holding. The Turbohaler™ trainer is used for training in the use of this device. It illuminates one, two or three lights when a patient achieves an inspiratory flow rate of greater than 20, 40 and 60 litres/minute respectively. Likewise, the Twisthaler™ trainer has been developed for training in the use of this device. The Mag-Flo™ is a device which has a green light indicator which turns on when the device is used correctly. One form of the Mag-Flo™ device can be used with the Clickhaler™, Twisthaler™ and other inhalers, and there is another with a different calibration which suits the Turbohaler™.

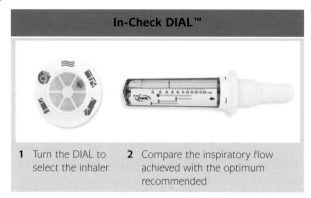

In-Check DIAL™

1 Turn the DIAL to select the inhaler

2 Compare the inspiratory flow achieved with the optimum recommended

Figure 39. The In-Check DIAL™.

The In-Check DIAL™ (see Figure 39) is a tool for training patients to produce the optimum inspiratory flow rate for a particular inhaler and in assessing their ability to use a particular device, as it can be used to simulate the inspiratory flow rate needed for a range of devices. The device consists of an inspiratory flow rate meter with a variable resistance. The resistances are calibrated to simulate the inspiratory flow rate resistance of the most commonly used devices, and a scale reflects the optimum inspiratory flow rate range for each device. Devices may be effective at flow rates outside these ranges, but the lung deposition will be affected.

It is important that a patient's ability to use a particular device is assessed both when they are well and when they are experiencing an exacerbation or their asthma is poorly controlled, as their ability to produce the optimum inspiratory flow rate may be affected by the state of their asthma at the time of testing.

Asthma action plans

Asthma education for patients includes the use of action plans. These are systematic sets of information and instructions which enable people with asthma, and their families, to recognize and self-manage exacerbations.

The use of personal written action plans by people with asthma is established as a way of improving care and outcome,[49,64,75–77] and their use is recommended in most national guidelines. Studies of patients practising self-monitoring in conjunction with use of a written action plan and regular medical review have found significantly fewer hospitalizations, emergency department visits and lost time from work. However, there is some controversy regarding the nature of action plans and their efficacy, particularly related to the use of written plans and routine PEF monitoring.

While there is controversy regarding the use of written versus verbal plans[64,78] and the use of peak flow combined with symptom plans versus symptom-only plans, it is generally agreed that patients should know when to adjust their medication and when to call for help. This can be achieved in different ways depending on the ability and aptitude of the patient. An action plan may range from a simple written instruction to the patient to see the doctor if symptoms become troublesome to a fully-fledged detailed, pre-printed written plan such as the examples in Figures 15 and 16.[79]

What patients need to know: anticipating uncontrolled asthma

People with asthma need to become familiar with the factors that trigger their symptoms (see Table 2). Medication can be adjusted or initiated before exposure to known triggers, and also when symptoms begin, such as during a viral infection. Studies on people who died from asthma show consistently that danger signs were present but not recognized by patients, their families or health professionals.

What patients need to know: when is asthma uncontrolled?

Two methods may be used to determine poor asthma control: first, recognition by the patients of exacerbations of symptoms and their response to treatment; second, changes in PEF (see Tables 25 and 26).

Symptoms (cough, wheeze, difficulty breathing):

- Reliever medication (short-acting β_2-agonist bronchodilators) should relieve symptoms and this effect should last for at least 4 hours.
- Patients should know that they must obtain medical assistance if either of these criteria are not met when taking reliever medication for exacerbations.

These patterns are depicted in Figures 40–42. The use of guidelines[81] on the charts may help patients identify when their asthma is uncontrolled. In these figures, a line has been drawn at 80%, 60% and 40% of the patient's best reading (500 litres/minute). Written instructions then advise the patient to increase or resume their inhaled steroid when

Table 25. Signs of uncontrolled asthma

Symptoms not responding to usual reliever medication

Relief medication not lasting for 4 hours

PEF varying or fluctuating

PEF dropping

Early morning dips in PEF

Table 26. Peak expiratory flow diary monitoring

There is considerable controversy regarding the use of PEF monitoring by patients. Some studies have demonstrated that patients are sometimes unreliable and non-compliant in using PEF charts,[80] while others highlight the value of using objective measurement in preventing asthma deaths.[3] In the authors' opinion, patients should be taught to recognize three patterns of uncontrolled asthma using PEF charts:

- Fluctuations in readings from day to day or day to evening
- Dropping readings
- Early morning dips

the readings drop below 80%, to initiate oral steroids when these are heading towards 60% and to seek urgent medical attention when the readings reach 40%.

What patients need to know: what to do when asthma is uncontrolled

The ultimate aim of self-management is to avoid asthma becoming uncontrolled; however, should the patient's symptoms and/or PEF indicate that an exacerbation is

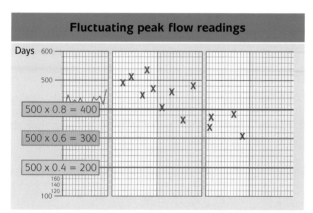

Figure 40. Fluctuating peak flow readings.

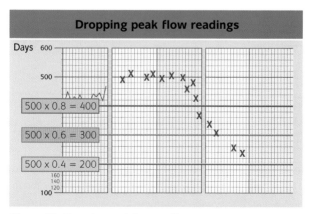

Figure 41. Dropping peak flow readings.

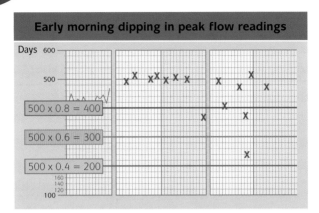

Figure 42. Early morning dipping in peak flow readings.

imminent, they should follow the guidelines provided by their doctor or nurse in their agreed asthma action plan. This might include initiating or increasing medication or simply an urgent instruction to seek medical advice. Although many health professionals provide their patients with a course of oral steroids, many are unaware that these take at least 6 hours to start working. Therefore, the earlier this medication is initiated the better. Patients not provided with medication for attacks should ensure they seek medical attention as soon as they realize their asthma is going out of control. Primary care receptionists need to be sympathetic to the needs of these patients and ensure that they are attended to urgently. Conversely, the patients themselves should be instructed to state, in these circumstances, that their asthma is out of control.

Compliance with medical advice on medication

The term compliance is used to describe the extent to which the patient's behaviour coincides with the advice offered by the health professional. Although it is still very much in current use, non-compliance has become a less fashionable term to use as it may imply a subservient relationship. A number of contemporary terms are used to encourage a more equal partnership between the patient and health care professional. These terms include concordance, adherence and therapeutic partnership. All of these terms assume the patient will make a decision about managing their asthma after discussion with the health care professional.

A number of studies have reviewed non-compliance rates. Non-compliance is a particular problem in the management of respiratory disease; Claxton *et al.*[82] found rates varied between 37% and 92% (mean of 55%). The European Community Respiratory Health Survey showed worldwide variation in compliance rates.[83] Where patients were asked if they normally take all the medications prescribed for their breathing, compliance rates were 40% in the USA, 65% in the UK and 78% in Iceland. When asked if they take all of their medication if they become symptomatic, the rate for patients from the UK increased to 77%.

A recent UK data analysis identified that 25% of asthma patients have compliance rates of less than 30%.[84] The economic implications of such a poor level of compliance can be judged from the estimation by the WHO that the economic costs for managing asthma are higher than those of managing HIV and tuberculosis combined.

Furthermore, non-compliance with advice or medication is a complex issue. Ley *et al.*[85] identified the variables that influence non-compliance. These subtypes include intentional non-compliance, unintentional non-compliance and constructive non-compliance:

- Intentional non-compliance – the patient makes a choice not to adhere to the treatment regimen; this may be because they do not agree with the diagnosis, they may deny they have the disease, or they may disagree with the treatment or advice they have been given.
- Unintentional non-compliance – the patient may have difficulty administering the medication.
- Constructive non-compliance – there is a valid reason for not adhering to the treatment regime; for example,

fear of side-effects from using steroids to control asthma symptoms, or because of the cost of the medications (patients may not be able to afford more than one inhaler and they then make a decision as to which one to purchase).

Non-compliance may result from many causes (Table 27) and usually involves the underuse of preventative medication, typically inhaled corticosteroids. This frequently leads to an overuse of reliever medication, an increase in acute exacerbations of asthma and may lead to an increased need for emergency intervention.

The model of health belief developed by Becker *et al.*[86,87] identified various reasons behind differing values and behaviour in health. These include age, gender and social class. People may attend with preconceived ideas regarding their disease. They may have a perception that their condition is more (or less) serious than is the fact. The patient may have a predetermined view of how the disease may be treated. For example, a patient may expect to be given an antibiotic for symptoms of asthma such as a cough and wheeze, where there is no evidence for such treatments unless specific infections are present. There may also be a prejudice against particular forms of treatment – for example, the continuous use of preventer therapy when asthma symptoms are intermittent. As described previously, a patient may also make a value judgement based on finance. To add to this, they may also be willing to pay for non-prescription medicines when effective medications are available without or at reduced cost on prescription. Information gained from the media, friends and family may also influence their decision-making process.

Health professionals should also understand that patients might not be necessarily concerned with gaining any improvement in their health. Reasons such as attention seeking or financial gain (e.g. disability benefit) may lead them to avoid treatment that will change their current health state.

Patients may also have either an unrealistic expectation of the level of improvement that can be attained or, more

Table 27. Factors that may contribute to non-compliance

Patient-related factors

Denial or acceptance of diagnosis

Patient belief and values

Misunderstanding of condition/treatment

Lack of family/social support

Peer group "pressure/opinion"

Anxiety over treatment/fear of side-effects

Preference for alternative therapies

Embarrassment

Forgetfulness

Adverse family circumstances

Language, reading or eyesight difficulties

Poor inhaler technique/unsuitable inhaler for individual ability

Adapt/adjust lifestyle to symptoms

Coexisting disease/morbidity

Treatment-related factors

Lack of noticeable benefit

Method of administration

Frequency of dosing

Complexity of regimen

Multiple prescription charges

Side-effects

Other factors

Mild intermittent symptoms

Poor communication between patient and health care provider

Dislike/distrust of health service

worryingly, may consider that their current state of health, with its impairment in quality of life, may be the best that can be achieved. One of the key findings in the AIRE study was that many patients with asthma have low expectations of the quality of life they can achieve. Among patients who considered that they were well, more than a third had daily symptoms of breathlessness, wheezing and chest tightness.[5]

Improving non-compliance

These factors can be identified with effective consultation and communication skills, although it is doubtful that complete compliance can ever be achieved[88] (see Table 28).

A prejudgement in terms of the health beliefs of a patient may lead to a misunderstanding of their needs, desires or intentions regarding the management of their

Table 28. Some questions which help encourage a discussion about compliance
How often do you forget to use your (add relevant preventer colour) inhaler?
How much benefit do you think you are getting from your inhaler?
How much does the inconvenience or embarrassment of taking your asthma medicines bother you?
Many patients have told me they find it difficult to take all their medicines exactly as prescribed. How hard is it for you?
During the last week, how often have you found it hard to take your medicine exactly as prescribed? .
What would you say are the least satisfactory/most satisfactory things about taking your medicine?
How could we make it easier for you to take your medicine as prescribed?
How much does the cost of your medicines bother you?
Do you have any concerns about taking your treatment?

asthma. This mismatch in perception can help explain why health professionals sometimes find patient behaviour difficult to understand.

It is clear from other studies that information alone does not influence compliance, and health professionals should be moving towards achieving joint agreement on management with the patient and, where appropriate, their carers.[89]

Many of the protocols for managing patient consultations have the understanding of patient expectations as a key element. However, if it is not taken into account that these expectations may be much lower than is realistic, then the success of any consultation may be reduced, potentially resulting in little change in the patient's asthma control.

For this first element of the consultation to be successful, the health professional must gain an understanding of the patient's agenda and ensure that their expectations regarding the outcome of the consultation are realistic and understood.

The patient's hopes and fears can be addressed and their expectations can be put into context. Only when this has been completed can real progress be made towards identifying the problem and gaining a common understanding through appropriate strategies. This approach through a common understanding should lead to better compliance/adherence/concordance with medication and health advice[5] (see Table 29).

Delivery of care

The number of people dying from asthma and the number of adults admitted to hospital because of their asthma have reduced over the past 10 years and this may have resulted in a sense of complacency that asthma is being well managed. A number of surveys have clearly demonstrated unchanging levels of asthma-related morbidity (see p. 10). Despite the availability of good and effective medications to control patients' symptoms, morbidity persists due to this disease, for which there are a number of possible explanations.

Table 29. Strategies for improving compliance

Treatment-related interventions

Provide clear instructions

Ensure patient understands the instructions

Simplify treatment

Review treatment to reduce number of doses without jeopardizing asthma control

Review and reinforce good inhaler technique

Reduce number of prescribed medications

Educational/psychological interventions

Build compliance objectives into the self-management plan

Educate the patient

Tailor level and amount of education to suit patient

Repeat educational messages for reinforcement

Written information/tapes/video for the patient to take away

Encourage patient to record medication use (e.g. in asthma diary)

Use lifestyle cues (e.g. tooth-brushing, meals) as reminders

Refer to patient support groups and, if appropriate, agencies for financial/social support   *(continued)*

People with asthma:
- may not be aware their symptoms are due to asthma, and think that these are simply "part of life" and accept them;
- may not appreciate that they have lifestyle limitations imposed by inadequately controlled asthma;
- may choose, for a variety of reasons, to live with these symptoms;
- may not be offered or attend for regular asthma review;
- may not get the opportunity to explain their concerns and symptoms when consulting a health professional;

Table 29 (continued). Strategies for improving compliance
General principles
Establish a positive, productive relationship
Understanding health benefits/fears
Make consultations patient-centred
Maintain regular contact with patient
Discover and address individual barriers to compliance
Address emotional as well as practical issues
Enable, don't impose
Involve family member/carer where possible
Remember that knowledge alone will not change behaviour
One or two changes at a time
Continually check patient understanding
Be consistent with your advice
Ensure primary care team members give the same advice
Development of a verbal contract between patient and health care provider

- may be taking an inadequate/inappropriate amount of therapy.

Asthma care may take place in either the primary or secondary sectors or as part of "shared care". Shared care consists of primary care and hospital staff working together with a structured clinical format to ensure continuity of care. This method of care may be appropriate for those individuals with a history of near fatal episodes, brittle asthma or those with a confirmed diagnosis and persistent symptoms. Those individuals with persistent symptoms should have specialist review to clarify the diagnosis.

Ideally, there should be a process of structured care in place for those individuals who have required emergency treatment, irrespective of whether this was in primary care, emergency room or through admission to hospital. This group may also benefit from critical event analysis of causal factors, compliance issues and education on self-management skills.

The provision of adequate care as outlined in evidence-based guidelines such as GINA[49] and the BTS/SIGN British Asthma Guidelines[35] affords guidance for health care system providers. Appropriately managed routine clinical review is effective in improving asthma control, reducing school and work absence and reducing exacerbation rates.[90]

Who delivers the care appears to be less important than how it is delivered. Depending on the health care system the review may take place with a doctor, nurse, pharmacist or other type of health care worker. The health professional carrying out the review should have a special interest and adequate training in asthma management. For example, it has been shown that targeting particular groups of patients through a nurse-run intervention can be effective at reducing morbidity.[91]

An asthma register should be established. How this is developed will depend on the resources available. Within the UK, most primary care practices are computerized and creating a list of people with a diagnosis of asthma should be straightforward. This list may be inaccurate to some degree and may, for example, contain patients with other diseases such as COPD. These patients may need a clinical review in order that they can be placed on the appropriate register. In the same way, other disease registers such as one of people with COPD may contain patients where the diagnosis should be asthma. Again, careful clinical review will help clarify the diagnosis. Once the asthma list has been generated, the basic register can be subdivided to give an active/inactive asthma register. In the UK, data entry is based on the hierarchical Read code system, which allows comprehensive recording and hence extraction facilities for audit and research. The General Practice Airways Group (GPIAG)[92] has developed a comprehensive list of Read codes to enable standardization of data entry for respiratory disease in primary care. The quality of data entry on general practice systems varies; this may be improved through the

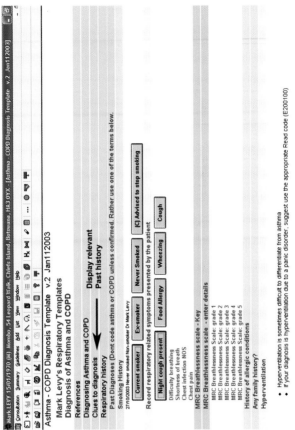

Figure 43. Computer data template for recording consultation data (Vision system).

use of data entry templates (see Figures 43 and 44). The process of developing and maintaining an accurate and up-to-date register takes time, but is worthwhile. As the register develops, a structured approach to clinical review can be formulated. A structured record card or computer template should incorporate a method for recording an adequate history and examination findings, including recordings of peak flows, inhaler technique, morbidity monitoring, treatment and planned actions. The use of these systems

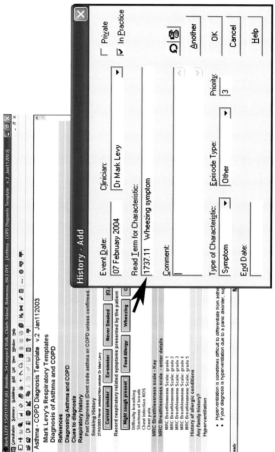

Figure 44. Computer data template for recording consultation data, showing the use of a "Button" to select the correct Read code for wheezing (Vision system).

may encourage self-management, assist the health professional as an "*aide-mémoire*" while also providing a useful audit tool. Effective communication and consultation skills are an essential ingredient of any review, as detailed in the section on compliance (see p. 94).

The provision of asthma care needs to be proactive, accessible, flexible and responsive to the asthma population that it serves. A number of people with chronic disease will, for a variety of reasons, still not avail themselves of the service for a routine review of their asthma; sadly, it is often the case that those people most requiring regular review are those who are least likely to attend. An alternative approach may be necessary, such as of the use of a routine telephone review of asthma.[93] In this study, there was no statistically significant difference in quality of life measurements or satisfaction between the group of patients seen in clinic or those reviewed by telephone. Clearly, peak flow and inhaler technique cannot be checked within this system of review, and therefore careful selection of suitable patients may be necessary. Another study, investigating the effect of patient education following hospital attendance for acute attacks of asthma, also utilized telephone follow-up for non-attendees. These patients had been previously taught how to use peak flow meters, and the readings were significantly better in the intervention group.[48] The most effective method of review should be selected for each individual patient. Health professionals should have heightened awareness for certain patient groups; these may include adolescents and young people, those with complex needs such as ethnic groups, the socially disadvantaged and those with learning disability or psychiatric disease.

The BTS/SIGN guidelines recommend identifying groups of patients at risk of developing near fatal or fatal asthma and targeting appropriate care (see Table 17). These people with asthma should remain under specialist supervision indefinitely.

Audit is an essential part of chronic disease management and regular audit will help identify any deficiencies in organizational as well as clinical aspects of the care provided. The BTS/SIGN guidelines have produced a list of audit points, which are useful for both the primary care and hospital clinics. The GPIAG website provides suggestions for auditing asthma care based on the British guidelines.[92] In order to ensure retrieval of good quality data, it is essential that data are entered consistently, ideally through the use of templates.[37]

Environmental Factors and Other Diseases

Occupational asthma

When diagnosing asthma in any adult, it is important to consider possible causes. Many general practitioners record information on their patients' occupations when they first join the practice. However, this information is not often related to subsequent diagnoses. In a study of general practice records to assess the overall burden of occupational asthma in the community, nearly a third of the patients with adult-onset asthma in the practice population were in jobs known to be significant causes of occupational asthma, yet a potential link between their occupation and symptoms had only been recorded in 18% of patients in these jobs.[94]

Occupational exposures account for about 10% of adult asthma. Unfortunately, many affected individuals remain undiagnosed; this may be due to difficulties in making this diagnosis, as well as reluctance to refer these patients from primary to secondary care. Occupational asthma is often a hidden disease. The individual may not admit the possibility of an occupational link for their symptoms for fear of losing their job. Early diagnosis is important because recovery is enhanced when an affected worker is removed from exposure within 12 months of first symptoms.

Diagnosis of occupational asthma follows essentially the same process as in the case of other adults with asthma, with the additional meticulous evaluation regarding aetiology. The history, in conjunction with objective measures demonstrating reversible airflow obstruction and response to treatment, all help in the process of diagnosis. There are two questions that may assist in establishing an occupational cause in patients with adult-onset asthma:

- Are you better on days away from work?
- Are you better on holiday?

Typically, symptoms of asthma due to occupational factors are worse on working days. The sufferer often wakes at night, and this improves when the person is away from work. As is the case with many people with asthma, sufferers from occupational asthma may experience symptoms triggered by exposure to various irritants such as dusts or fumes.

The diagnosis of work-related asthma needs to be confirmed objectively. This can be done by carrying out pulmonary function tests at work and off work. Two-hourly peak flow charts may be helpful. However, some patients with occupational asthma may have normal lung function as well as negative skin tests.

The occupational physician may also do challenge tests, where lung function is measured before and after exposure to suspected agents.

In considering cases for compensation as well as future work environments, two further questions need to be asked, ideally by a specialist in occupational medicine:

- Has the person's asthma been worsened or aggravated by exposure to occupational factors?
- Has the asthma been caused by exposure to occupational factors?

Physicians and patients seeking information on occupational asthma may find the Oasys and Occupational Asthma website useful.[95]

Rhinitis and asthma

Combined allergic rhinitis and asthma syndrome (CARAS)

Allergic rhinitis and allergic asthma frequently coexist in patients.[96,97] There is current debate whether these diseases are part of the same clinical condition, and there is also discussion on possible terminology to be used for this condition. Experts currently favour the term "Combined Allergic Rhinitis and Asthma Syndrome" or CARAS. CARAS is defined as patients who have "concurrent clinical or subclinical upper and lower respiratory tract symptoms".

The upper and lower airways are functionally linked, so it seems logical that patients may suffer from rhinitis as well as asthma. However, patients diagnosed with one of these conditions are often under-diagnosed for the other. Therefore, it is important to consider rhinitis in all patients with asthma and similarly asthma in all patients diagnosed with rhinitis. People suffering from atopic dermatitis or rhinitis may later develop asthma or, in other words, may be "at risk" of developing asthma.[98] However, these people may in fact be in the early stages of CARAS. In patients with rhinitis and asthma, it is essential to take a detailed history to exclude aspirin-sensitive asthma.

There are various links being researched between upper and lower airway function and theoretical mechanisms of CARAS. These include mouth breathing, due to nasal blockage in rhinitis, which leads to inhalation of cold air and allergens, due to the loss of warming and filtration in the nose, with resultant bronchoconstriction. In addition, various immunological mechanisms, including allergen activation of IgE in sensitized individuals with nasal symptoms as well as bronchoconstriction and hypersecretion of mucus, are being researched.

Treatment for CARAS should be directed at the underlying inflammatory processes common to allergic rhinitis and asthma. This includes intranasal glucocorticosteroids, antihistamines and H1 antagonists, which in various combinations have improved rhinitis as well as asthma morbidity.

In children, upper respiratory infections and asthma exacerbations can be controlled by continuous antihistamine treatment. In the ETAC (Early Treatment of the Atopic Child) study, continuous antihistamine treatment has been shown to reduce the number of at-risk children who subsequently develop asthma.[45]

Antibiotic therapy for chronic sinusitis in children has been shown to improve lower airway symptoms. Sometimes surgical intervention may help in controlling asthma in patients with either nasal polyposis or rhinosinusitis and asthma.

Uncontrolled allergic rhinitis can lead to worsening of coexisting asthma. Prompt and effective treatment of nasal disease can have a marked beneficial effect on preventing the development of asthma[45] and on existing asthma symptoms. A recent review identified two studies on outcomes of treatment of allergic rhinitis in patients with asthma, and concluded that this reduces utilization of acute health care services due to asthma.[99]

Most guidelines include warnings that patients with concomitant allergic rhinitis and asthma may be prescribed excess inhaled steroids. Therefore, prescribers should ensure that the total dose of corticosteroid does not exceed recommended levels.

Specialist treatment such as immunotherapy may be helpful in patients with CARAS.

Aspirin-sensitive asthma

The prevalence of aspirin-sensitive asthma (also referred to as aspirin-induced/intolerant asthma) is difficult to estimate and different studies suggest that between 1% and 20% of the adult asthma population is affected.[100] It is probably under-diagnosed and may be under-reported, as people with asthma may deliberately avoid the use of aspirin and non-steroidal anti-inflammatory drugs (NSAIDs) because of adverse reactions. Patients and indeed health professionals may fail to make the connection between aspirin use and symptoms. Aspirin-intolerant asthma occurs in adults, usually in their third decade, and is more common in females.

Aspirin-sensitive asthma presents with a distinctive clinical picture.[101] The history is of worsening asthma after ingestion of aspirin or NSAID, causing mucosal inflammatory disease within hours of their use. The individual will have a history of asthma, rhinitis symptoms, nasal polyps or possibly sinus disease. The asthma is often difficult to control.

Skin-prick tests to aspirin are always negative. Diagnosis can only be confirmed using an aspirin challenge test, which must be done in a controlled environment, with available resuscitation facilities. More recently, the measurement of urinary LTE_4 has accompanied these tests. Blood and airway eosinophils are increased.

The mechanism of action of aspirin is due to inhibition of the enzyme cyclo-oxygenase (COX). This enzyme plays a key role in the generation of prostaglandins from arachidonic acid. This results in an imbalance of pro-inflammatory leukotrienes. Individuals who produce increased levels of cysteinyl leukotrienes have an increase risk of developing aspirin-intolerant asthma.

The BTS/SIGN guidelines[35] state that there is a theoretical reason to treat people with aspirin-sensitive asthma with leukotriene receptor antagonists. However, they advise that at present there is little evidence to suggest that aspirin-sensitive asthma should be treated in any different way to asthma generally, other than avoidance of aspirin and NSAIDs.

Asthma in pregnancy

The goals for managing asthma in pregnancy are to maintain the well-being of both the mother and the foetus. This can be achieved by optimizing preventative therapy, regular review of asthma control, and close liaison between the obstetrician and health professional responsible for asthma care. It has been suggested that, during pregnancy, one-third of women will suffer deterioration in asthma control, one-third will have an improvement and one-third will have asthma that remains unchanged. Those women with severe asthma are likely to have worsening asthma during pregnancy.[102]

Reduced peak flow recordings have been demonstrated in pre-menstrual women who have asthma, and some women may actually present at these times with clinical symptoms of asthma. It is suggested, although the mechanism has not been defined, that a drop in oestradiol and progesterone may be responsible. On the other hand, oestradiol, progesterone and cortisol levels increase in pregnancy but do not necessarily result in improved asthma control. The respiratory physiological changes alter some aspects of lung function but dynamic lung volumes remain unchanged. Therefore, if changes do occur in the FEV_1 and FVC or FEV_1/FVC ratio, this generally indicates poorly controlled asthma.

It is important not to confuse the normal physiological changes that occur during pregnancy as uncontrolled asthma. Rhinitis-type symptoms may occur and it is normal to have shortness of breath or an increased sensation of breathing during the last trimester.

The highest risk to the mother and the foetus is that of uncontrolled asthma and attacks, and the risk that asthma poses in pregnancy is clearly greatest in women with severe asthma or obstetric complications. However, foetal distress can occur even when there is no maternal hypoxia, as the maternal compensatory mechanism will maintain the blood flow and oxygenation of the maternal organs as a priority.

The therapeutic management of asthma should be optimized using inhaled corticosteroids and β_2-agonist bronchodilators, following the same stepwise guidance as with non-pregnant patients of the same age and asthma severity. Oral steroids are indicated for uncontrolled asthma as they are in the non-pregnant patient and in fact may be life-saving therapy. The BTS/SIGN[35] guidelines at present recommend leukotriene antagonists should not be commenced during pregnancy, as data on their safety are limited. However, the guidelines suggest that if the woman is already taking them and they are beneficial they should be continued.

During labour and whilst breast feeding, women should continue to take their normal medication. It is reassuring to note that exacerbations during labour are rare.

The Future

A number of factors have improved and influenced asthma care in the past. These include:

- Better understanding of the mechanisms of asthma.
- Increased range of medications to manage asthma.
- National and international guidelines for asthma.
- Specific training for health professionals in asthma care.

However, surveys have clearly demonstrated that there remains a high level of asthma morbidity and mortality.

Current deficiencies in asthma care include:

- Inadequate services to deliver asthma care.
- Provision of care by generalist health professionals who may not have sufficient skills to manage a chronic disease.
- Insufficient use of personal asthma action plans – patients are ill-equipped for the task of self-management.
- Poor identification of patients who are not adhering to or unable to comply with medical advice (i.e. who may not be taking their medication regularly, who are unable to use their inhaler or who are unable to recognize deteriorating asthma).
- Many patients still suffer despite maximum medication. Do we have the right medications for asthma?

Research on asthma deaths has identified that most deaths were avoidable. Perhaps a more proactive approach is required in the future, through enabling patients by teaching self-management skills and providing action plans for people with asthma, while targeting specific high-risk patients.

Patient-focused care, with personalized asthma action plans, is one of the most effective interventions for adults and children in the routine management of asthma.[103] For patient-focused care to be effective, a partnership between health professionals and their patients is essential. Good communication and a mutual understand of each other's expectations is critical to achieve a successful outcome. Studies have shown that many patients experience a heavy burden of symptoms. Some health professionals measure asthma control based purely on signs and symptoms, whereas the patients tend to focus on being "able or unable" to do normal daily activities.[104] Expert patient programmes, recently developed in the UK, aim to ensure that patients have the know-how to manage everyday aspects of their health and condition.[89]

Scientists are working to understand the complex immunological and inflammatory mechanisms underlying asthma. While the complex interactions between the cells, chemical mediators and airway nerves are better understood and many individual cells and cytokines have been identified, the importance of each and their interactions are yet to be understood. When this has been achieved, we will perhaps be able to identify different subgroups of asthma to target specific drugs.

Many developments have occurred to identify new therapies for the management of asthma. Research has focused on the development of specific blockers of various parts of the inflammatory cascade, but most of the products developed, some of which have produced promising results *in vitro*, have been disappointing in clinical research.

Several anti-IgE monoclonal antibody classes of drugs are in early or full development. One of these, the injectable drug "omalizumab", has been shown in clinical trials to be effective in improving lung function and asthma symptoms. It is likely to be restricted at present to patients with severe asthma who do not respond to current preventer treatments.[105]

Ciclesonide is a novel inhaled glucocoticosteroid under clinical development. It is activated in the lung and has a high affinity to the glucocorticoid receptor. Studies suggest it might have less systemic side-effects.[106]

Alongside drug development, researchers are striving to improve inhaled delivery systems. A large proportion of the aerosolized drug is swallowed, with the potential to cause side-effects without any beneficial clinical effect. In an attempt to address this, research is being undertaken into the development of mono-dispersed particles. By dropping liquids onto a form of spinning wheel, particles of a predetermined size can be produced. Metered dose inhalers containing such liquids have been shown to have a greater clinical effect per actuation than those containing a normal mix of particle sizes. This has potential in terms of reducing the quantity of drug needed for clinical effect, and therefore the potential for side-effects.

Finally, the way we measure asthma control may advance with the introduction of measuring nitric oxide concentration in exhaled breath. The measurement of exhaled nitric oxide is a non-invasive objective measurement of airway inflammation and the effectiveness of anti-inflammatory drugs.

Frequently Asked Questions

What is asthma?

Asthma is a chronic inflammatory disorder of the airways with reversible obstruction. Susceptible individuals may have a variety of symptoms, none of which are specific for asthma. These may include wheeze, cough, shortness of breath and chest tightness. With asthma these symptoms tend to be intermittent, variable, often worse at night and, for allergic asthma, provoked by trigger factors.

Why is asthma so common?

The prevalence of asthma throughout the world is increasing, especially in industrialized countries. The cause of this is unknown, but is thought to be a combination of predisposing factors (e.g. atopy) and environmental factors. These environmental factors may include lifestyle, diet and pollution.

Why are people still dying from asthma?

Many deaths due to asthma involve avoidable factors. These include failure to recognize danger signs by patients, their relatives and health professionals. Poor adherence to medical advice, inadequate treatment, insufficient monitoring and not recognizing deteriorating asthma all contribute to these deaths.

Why do people have allergic responses?

The allergic response is not necessarily a bad thing. In fact, it is an allergic response by IgE synthesis, making the gut hostile to parasitic infestation (perhaps more relevant nowadays in developing countries). As the lung is derived from the gut during the embryonic stage, it is perhaps understandable why the same response occurs in a sensitive individual when exposed to a specific trigger. This response, in the lung, to an inappropriate target such as house dust mites leads to the symptoms of asthma.

How are allergens identified?
Allergens are identified by careful history taking and may be confirmed by skin-prick testing to aeroallergens, the measurement of allergen-specific IgE (sIgE) in cases of suspected food allergy and helped by serial peak flow measurement in the workplace if an occupational allergen is suspected.

Should any medication be avoided?
β-Blockers, including eye drops, are contraindicated for anybody with a diagnosis of asthma. Aspirin and non-steroidal anti-inflammatory drugs (NSAIDs) should be used with caution in people with asthma. Any history of worsening symptoms following their use is an indication that they should be avoided.

How is recurrent wheezing in the under 2s managed?
Causes include pathologically small airways, viral infections or asthma. After a detailed history and examination, if the probable diagnosis is asthma then a trial of therapy, including inhaled corticosteroids, and monitor response is appropriate. If the diagnosis is unclear, or after a trial of therapy with no response, consider referral for specialist opinion.

Do children grow out of asthma?
Many do, however many do not! Therefore, it is very important that patients as well as health professionals should be aware of their past medical history. In many people, their asthma goes into remission, sometimes for years, only for the condition to recur later in life.

What are the benefits of inhaled corticosteroids?
Inhaled corticosteroids are the most effective long-term medication for persistent asthma. They reduce airway hyper-responsiveness, reduce symptoms, prevent exacerbations

and improve peak flow. Inhaled corticosteroids should be administered commensurate with the severity of disease.

What are the risks of taking inhaled corticosteroid therapy?

Common side-effects include dysphonia and oral candidiasis. There appears to be little evidence that doses below 800 mcg (BDP equivalent) total daily dose cause any short-term effects in adults. However, there is a possibility of dose-related reduction of bone density. Doses above 400 mcg (BDP equivalent) have been shown to induce short-term growth suppression and adrenal suppression in children, and therefore referral to a specialist is advised if these doses are necessary in children. Furthermore, effort should be taken to reduce the dose to the lowest required for maintaining disease control.

What are the risks of taking short-acting β_2-agonist bronchodilator therapy?

Common side-effects include short-term tremor, tachycardia and transient headache. These may occur when somebody starts using this class of drug or if they are used frequently or in high dose. Generally, these drugs are very safe.

Should inhaled corticosteroids be stopped when a course of prednisolone is started in acute asthma?

It is generally agreed that the inhaled corticosteroid should be continued when an occasional short course of prednisolone is required to control an exacerbation. The main reason is to ensure continued compliance with inhaled therapy.

Is there a place for antibiotic therapy in exacerbations of asthma?

No, unless there are clear indications of an infection.

What is the difference between asthma and COPD?

COPD mainly occurs in people over 35 years old who smoke. Both conditions cause airway narrowing and airway limitation. Different cell types are involved in the patterns of inflammation in asthma and COPD. In COPD the narrowing is fixed with very little reversibility. In asthma the narrowing varies from day to day and there is a good degree of reversibility, either spontaneously or with anti-asthma medication. Spirometry is necessary for diagnosing COPD. Management of the two conditions is different and therefore appropriate investigations are necessary to make the diagnosis.

Is peak flow monitoring important?

Yes, for confirming the diagnosis, self-monitoring and during attacks. As part of a personalized asthma action plan, peak flow monitoring can enhance self-management. However, the patient needs to be willing to accept the need to monitor peak flow. It may take time and encouragement for confidence to develop so that they are able to interpret the results and implement appropriate self-management strategies. Peak flow monitoring is an essential part of assessing the severity and duration of an asthma exacerbation; this is helpful in deciding when to discontinue oral steroid medication for these events.

How often should asthma be reviewed?

In primary care, proactive structured clinical assessment should take place every 3–12 months – if the patient agrees to attend! More frequent assessment is needed (every 1–3 months) in severe patients, and daily following acute attacks. Seasonal reviews may be more appropriate in those with asthma during these periods. This may take place within the consultation room or by telephone.

How do I know when to call for help?

People who have asthma should be advised to call for help if their symptoms get worse (cough, breathlessness, wheeze or tight chest). They should also call for help if they become too breathless to talk, or their reliever (short-acting β_2-agonist bronchodilator) inhaler does not help.

How can I tell if asthma is well controlled and can therefore decrease medication?

Asthma can be regarded as well controlled when there is no interference with normal daily activity or sleep disturbance and serial peak flow readings are stable. Assuming inhaled corticosteroids are used as prescribed and bronchodilator therapy is required on a very occasional basis, it would be appropriate to slowly reduce the inhaled corticosteroids. Decreasing the dose by 25–50% every 3 months should be considered whilst monitoring for any deteriorating symptoms.

References

1. The British Thoracic Society. *The Burden of Lung Disease*. A Statistics Report from the British Thoracic Society. www.brit-thoracic.org.uk, 13 November 2001. Last accessed on 30 November 2003.

2. Respiratory Alliance. Bridging the gap: commissioning and delivering high quality integrated respiratory healthcare. www.gpiag.org/news/bridging.php, 2003. Last accessed on 30 November 2003.

3. Bucknall CE, Slack R, Godley CC *et al.* Scottish Confidential Inquiry into Asthma Deaths (SCIAD), 1994–6. *Thorax* 1999; **54**(11): 978–984.

4. National Heart, Lung, and Blood Institute (NHLBI) (Bethesda). International consensus report on the diagnosis and treatment of asthma. *Eur Respir J* 1992; **5**: 601–641.

5. Rabe KF, Vermeire PA, Maier *et al*. Clinical management of asthma in 1999: the Asthma Insights and Reality in Europe (AIRE) study. *Eur Respir J* 2000; **16**: 802–807.

6. European Community Respiratory Health Survey. Variations in the prevalance of respiratory symptoms, self-reported asthma attacks, and use of asthma medication in the European Community Respiratory Health Survey (ECRHS). *Eur Respir J* 1996; **9**: 687–695.

7. The International Study of Asthma and Allergies in Childhood (ISAAC) Steering Committee. Worldwide variations in the prevelance of asthma symptoms: the International Study of Asthma and Allergies in Childhood. *Eur Respir J* 1998; **12**: 315–335.

8. Masoli M, Fabian D, Holt S *et al. Global Burden of Asthma*. Global Initiative for Asthma, 2003 (in press).

9. National Asthma Campaign Asthma Audit 2001. *Asthma J* 2001; **6**(Special Suppl 3).

10. Haahtela T, Lindholm H, Bjorksten F *et al*. Prevalence of asthma in Finnish young men. *Br Med J* 1990; **301**(6746): 266–268.

11. Aberg N, Hesselmar B, Aberg B *et al.* Increase of asthma, allergic rhinitis and eczema in Swedish school children between 1979 and 1991. *Clin Exp Allergy* 1995; **25**(9): 815–819.

12. Nakagomi T, Itaya H, Tominaga T *et al.* Is atopy increasing? *Lancet* 1994; **343:** 121–122.

13. Rona RJ, Chinn S, Burney PG. Trends in the prevalence of asthma in Scottish and English primary school children 1982–92. *Thorax* 1995; **50:** 992–993.

14. Omran M, Russell G. Continuing increase in respiratory symptoms and atopy in Aberdeen school children. *Br Med J* 1996; **312:** 34.

15. Asthma – United States, 1982–1992. *Morb Mortal Week Rep* 1995; **43**: 952–955. www.cdc.gov/mmwr/pdf/wk/mm4351.pdf. Last accessed on 11 February 2004.

16. Shaw RA, Crane J, O'Donnell TV *et al.* Increasing asthma prevalence in a rural New Zealand adolescent population: 1975–89. *Arch Dis Child* 1990; **65:** 1319–1323.

17. Peat JK. Changes in the prevalence of asthma and allergy in Australian children 1982–1992. *Am Rev Respir Dis* 1993; **147:** A800.

18. Sears MR, Greene JM, Willan AR *et al.* A longitudinal, population-based, cohort study of childhood asthma followed to adulthood. *New Engl J Med* 2003; **349**(15): 1414–1422.

19. World Health Organization (WHO). Bronchial asthma. WHO Fact Sheet No. 206. www.who.int/inf-fs/en/fact206.html. Last accessed on 23 November 2003.

20. Burke W, Fesinmeyer M, Reed K *et al*. Family history as a predictor of asthma risk. *Am J Prevent Med* 2003; **24**(2): 160–169.

21. Kurukulaaratchy RJ, Matthews S, Waterhouse L *et al.* Factors influencing symptom expression in children with bronchial hyperresponsiveness at 10 years of age – 1. *J Allergy Clin Immunol* 2003; **112**(2): 311–316.

22. Holgate ST, Church MK, Howarth PH *et al*. Genetic and environmental influences on airway inflammation in asthma [Review – 35 refs]. *Int Arch Allergy Immunol* 1995; **107**(1–3): 29–33.

23. Arshad SH, Stevens M, Hide DW. The effect of genetic and environmental factors on the prevalence of allergic disorders at the age of two years. *Clin Exp Allergy* 1994; **23**(6): 504–511.

24. Korppi M, Reijonen T, Poysa L *et al.* A 2- to 3-year outcome after bronchiolitis. *Am J Dis Children* 1993; **147**(6): 628–631.

25. Wilson NM. Virus infections, wheeze and asthma. *Paed Respir Rev* 2003; **4**(3): 184–192.

26. Busse WW, Rosenwasser LJ. Mechanisms of asthma. *J Allergy Clin Immunol* 2003; **111**(3, Part 2): S799–S804.

27. Bardana J. Occupational asthma and allergies. *J Allergy Clin Immunol* 2003; **111**(2, Part 3): 530–539.

28. Charlton I, Jones K, Bain J. Delay in diagnosis of childhood asthma and its influence on respiratory consultation rates. *Arch Dis Childhood* 1991; **66**(5): 633–635.

29. Jones A, Sykes AP. The effect of symptom presentation on delay in asthma diagnosis in children in a general practice. *Respir Med* 1990; **84**: 139–142.

30. Levy M, Bell L. General practice audit of asthma in childhood. *Br Med J* 1984; **289**(6452): 1115–1116.

31. Levy M. Delay in diagnosing asthma – is the nature of general practice to blame? *J Roy Coll Gen Pract* 1986; **36**(283): 52–53.

32. Tudor-Hart J. Wheezing in young children: problems of measurement and management. *J Roy Coll Gen Pract* 1986; **36**: 78–81.

33. Dennis SM, Price J, Vickers MR *et al.* The management of newly identified asthma in primary care in England. *Primary Care Respir J* 2002; **11**(4): 120–123.

34. Toop LJ. Active approach to recognising asthma in general practice. *Br Med J* 1985; **290**: 1629–1631.

35. BTS/SIGN. British guidelines on the management of asthma. *Thorax* 2003; **58**(Suppl 1): i1–i94.

36. Levy M, Hilton S. *Asthma in Practice*, 4th edn. London: Royal College of General Practitioners, 2000; pp. 9–112.

37. Levy M. Electronic patient records in asthma consultations: coding and datasets. *The Airways J* 2003; **1**: 85–87.

38. GPIAG. Diagnosis of asthma. www.gpiag.org/opinions/Opinion10.pdf, 28 November 2003. Last accessed on 28 November 2003.

39. Bellia V, Pistelli R, Filippazzo G *et al*. Prevalence of nocturnal asthma in a general population sample: determinants and effect of aging. *J Asthma* 2000; **37**(7): 595–602.

40. Dow L. The epidemiology and therapy of airflow limitation in the elderly. *Drugs Ageing* 1992; **2**(6): 546–559.

41. Bellia V, Battaglia S, Catalano F *et al*. Aging and disability affect misdiagnosis of COPD in elderly asthmatics: the SARA study. *Chest* 2003; **123**(4): 1066–1072.

42. National Institutes of Health, NHLBI. Global Initiative for Chronic Obstructive Lung Disease. Global Strategy for the Diagnosis, Management, and Prevention of Chronic Obstructive Pulmonary Disease (updated 2003). www.goldcopd.com/, 2001.

43. Martinez FD. Toward asthma prevention – does all that really matters happen before we learn to read? [comment]. *New Engl J Med* 2003; **349**(15): 1473–1475.

44. Woodcock A, Forster L, Matthews E *et al*. Control of exposure to mite allergen and allergen-impermeable bed covers for adults with asthma. *New Engl J Med* 2003; **349**(3): 225–236.

45. Warner JO. A double-blinded, randomized, placebo-controlled trial of cetirizine in preventing the onset of asthma in children with atopic dermatitis: 18 months' treatment and 18 months' posttreatment follow-up (ETAC). *J Allergy Clin Immunol* 2001; **108**(6): 929–937.

46. Strachan DP, Cook DG. Health effects of passive smoking. Parental smoking and childhood asthma: longitudinal and case control studies. *Thorax* 1998; **53**: 204–212.

47. Strachan DP. Hay fever, hygiene, and household size. *Br Med J* 1989; **299**: 1259–1260.

48. Levy ML, Robb M, Allen J *et al*. A randomized controlled evaluation of specialist nurse education following accident and

emergency department attendance for acute asthma. *Respir Med* 2000; **94**(9): 900–908.

49. Global Initiative for Asthma. *Pocket Guide for Asthma Management and Prevention* (summary of patient care information for primary health care professionals, NIH Publication No. 02-3659A). www.ginasthma.com/, 1 June 2002. Last accessed on 28 November 2003.

50. Guyatt GH, Juniper EF, Griffith LE *et al.* Children and adult perceptions of childhood asthma. *Pediatrics* 1997; **99**(2): 165–168.

51. Juniper EF, Guyatt GH, Ferrie PJ *et al.* Measuring quality of life in asthma. *Am Rev Respir Dis* 1993; **147**(4): 832–838.

52. Anie KA, Jones PW, Hilton SR *et al.* A computer-assisted telephone interview technique for assessment of asthma morbidity and drug use in adult asthma. *J Clin Epidemiol* 1996; **49**(6): 653–656.

53. Jones PW, Quirke FH, Bavestock CM *et al.* A self complete measure of health status for chronic airflow limitation. The St. Georges Respiratory questionnaire. *Am Rev Respir Dis* 1992; **145**: 1321–1327.

54. Jones PW. Quality of life, symptoms and pulmonary function in asthma: long-term treatment with nedocromil sodium examined in a controlled multicentre trial. Nedocromil Sodium Quality of Life Study Group. *Eur Respir J* 1994; **7**(1): 55–62.

55. Pearson MG, Bucknall CE, editors. *Measuring Clinical Outcome in Asthma: A Patient Focused Approach.* Royal College of Physicians, Clinical Effectiveness & Evaluation Unit, 1999.

56. Mohan G, Harrison BD, Badminton RM *et al.* A confidential enquiry into deaths caused by asthma in an English health region: implications for general practice [see comments]. *Br J Gen Pract* 1996; **46**(410): 529–532.

57. Calpin C, Macarthur C, Stephens D *et al*. Effectiveness of prophylactic inhaled steroids in childhood asthma: a systemic review of the literature. *J Allergy Clin Immunol* 1997; **100**: 452–457.

58. Adams NP, Bestall JB, Jones PW. Inhaled beclomethasone versus placebo for chronic asthma (Cochrane Review). The Cochrane Library No. 3, 2001.

59. Greening AP, Ind PW, Northfield M *et al.* Added salmeterol versus higher-dose corticosteroid in asthma patients with symptoms on existing inhaled corticosteroid. Allen & Hanburys Limited UK Study Group [see comments]. *Lancet* 1994; **344**(8917): 219–224.

60. Pauwels RA, Lofdahl CG, Postma DS *et al*. Effect of inhaled formoterol and budesonide on exacerbations of asthma. Formoterol and Corticosteroids Establishing Therapy (FACET) International Study Group [see comments]. *New Engl J Med* 1997; **337**(20): 1405–1411 [published erratum appears in *New Engl J Med* 1998; **338**(2):139].

61. O'Connor B, Bonnaud G, Haahtela T *et al*. Dose-ranging study of mometasone furoate dry powder inhaler in the treatment of moderate persistent asthma using fluticasone propionate as an active comparator. *Ann Allergy Asthma Immunol* 2001; **86**(4): 397–404.

62. Bousquet J, D'Urzo A, Hebert J *et al*. Comparison of the efficacy and safety of mometasone furoate dry powder inhaler to budesonide Turbuhaler. *Eur Respir J* 2000; **16**(5): 808–816.

63. Bernstein DI, Berkowitz RB, Chervinsky P *et al*. Dose-ranging study of a new steroid for asthma: mometasone furoate dry powder inhaler. *Respir Med* 1999; **93**(9): 603–612.

64. Holt S, Masoli M, Beasley R. The use of the self-management plan system of care in adult asthma. *Primary Care Respir J* 2004; **13**(1):19–27.

65. Global Initiative for Asthma (GINA). *Pocket Guide for Asthma Management and Prevention*. NIH Publication No. 02-3659A, 2002.

66. Gibson PG. Asthma action plans: use it or lose it. *Primary Care Resp J* 2004; **13:** 17–18.

67. Fleming DM, Sunderland R, Cross KW *et al.* Declining incidence of episodes of asthma: a study of trends in new episodes presenting to general practitioners in the period 1989–98. *Thorax* 2000; **55**(8): 657–661.

68. Levy ML. Assessment chart for acute asthma in primary care. www.gpiag.org/clinical/index.php, 2003. Last accessed on 28 November 2003.

69. Pearce L. Revisiting inhaler devices: selecting an inhaler. *Practice Nursing* 2002; **13**(12): 82.

70. Brocklebank D, Ram FS, Wright J. Comparison of the effectiveness of inhaler devices in asthma and chronic obstructive airways disease: a systematic review of the literature. *Health Technol Assess Rep* 2001; **5**: 1–149.

71. Pearce L. Do health professionals have sufficient knowledge and skill to teach optimum inspiratory flow (oif)? A study using the In-Check dial™ (icd) to evaluate inspiratory technique. *Am J Respir Crit Care Med* 2002; **165**(8): B3.

72. Barry PW, O'Callaghan C. Multiple actuations of salbutamol MDI into a spacer device reduce the amount of drug recovered in the respirable range. *Eur Respir J* 1994; **7**: 1707–1709.

73. Pierart F, Devadason SG, Wildhaber JH *et al.* Minimising electrostatic charge on a plastic spacer by use of ionic detergent. *Eur Respir J* 1997; **10**(Suppl 25): 220s.

74. Cates C. Holding chambers versus nebulisers for beta-agonist treatment of acute asthma. Cochrane Database of Systematic Reviews No. 2, 2001.

75. Gibson PG. Monitoring the patient with asthma: an evidence-based approach [Review – 72 refs]. *J Allergy Clin Immunol* 2000; **106**(1, Part 1): 17–26.

76. Gibson PG, Powell H, Coughlan J *et al.* Self-management education and regular practitioner review for adults with asthma [Review – 94 refs]. Cochrane Database of Systematic Reviews 2003; No. 1: CD001117 [update of Cochrane Database of Systematic Reviews 2000; No. 2: CD001117; PMID: 10796600].

77. Rachelefsky GS, Lewis CE, de la Sota A *et al.* Act (asthma care training) for kids. A childhood asthma self-management program. *Chest* 1985; **87**(1, Suppl): 98S–100S.

78. Toelle BG, Peat JK, Salome CM *et al.* Evaluation of a community-based asthma management program in a population sample of schoolchildren. *Med J Australia* 1993; **158**: 742–746.

79. National Asthma Campaign. NAC Self Management Plan. www.asthma.org.uk/about/pdf/control.pdf.

80. Turner MO, Taylor D, Bennett R *et al.* A randomized trial comparing peak expiratory flow and symptom self-management plans for patients with asthma attending a primary care clinic. *Am J Resp Crit Care Med* 1998; **157**(2): 540–546.

81. Hayward SA, Levy M. Patient self-management of asthma [letter]. *Br J Gen Pract* 1990; **40**(333): 166.

82. Claxton AJ, Cramer J, Pierce C. A systematic review of the associations between dose regimens and medication compliance. *Clin Ther* 2001; **23**(8): 1296–1310.

83. Cerveri I, Locatelli F, Zoia MC *et al.* International variations in asthma treatment compliance: the results of the European Community Respiratory Health Survey (ECRHS). *Eur Respir J* 1999; **14**(2): 288–294.

84. Das GR, Guest JF. Factors affecting UK primary-care costs of managing patients with asthma over 5 years. *Pharmacoeconomics* 2003; **21**(5): 357–369.

85. Ley P, Bradshaw PW, Eaves D *et al.* A method for increasing patients' recall of information presented by doctors. *Psychol Med* 1973; **3**(2): 217–220.

86. Becker MH. *Understanding Patient Compliance: The Contributions of Attitudes and Other Psychosocial Factors. New Directions in Patient Compliance*. New York: Lexington Books, 1979.

87. Eraker SA, Kirscht JP, Becker MH. Understanding and improving patient compliance [Review – 169 refs]. *Ann Intern Med* 1984; **100**(2): 258–268.

88. Pearce L. Asthma: the challenge of asthma treatment compliance. *Practice Nurse Supplement*, 1999.

89. Department of Health. The expert patient: a new approach to chronic disease management for the 21st century. www.doh.gov.uk/healthinequalities/ep_report.pdf, 20 November 2003.

90. Charlton I, Charlton G, Broomfield J *et al.* Audit of the effect of a nurse run asthma clinic on workload and patient morbidity in a general practice. *Br J Gen Pract* 1991; **41**: 227–231.

91. Dickerson J, Hutton S, Atkin A *et al*. Reducing asthma morbidity in the community: the effect of a targeted nurse-run asthma clinic in an English general practice. *Respir Med* 1997; **91**: 634–640.

92. Levy ML, Danzig L. General Practice Airways Group (GPIAG). www.gpiag.org, 28 November 2003. General Practitioners in Asthma Group. Last accessed on 28 November 2003.

93. Pinnock H, Bawden R, Proctor S *et al*. Accessibility, acceptability, and effectiveness in primary care of routine telephone review of asthma: pragmatic, randomised controlled trial. *Br Med J* 2003; **326**(7387): 477–479.

94. de Bono J, Hudsmith L. Occupational asthma: a community based study. *Occupational Med (Oxford)* 1999; **49**(4): 217–219.

95. Oasys Research Group (part of the Midland Thoracic Society for Occupational Asthma. www.occupationalasthma.com.

96. Robinson SM, Harrison BDW, Lambert MA. Effect of a preprinted form on the management of acute asthma in an accident and emergency department. *J Accid Emerg Med* 1996; **13**(2): 93–97.

97. Leynaert B, Neukirch F, Demoly P *et al*. Epidemiologic evidence for asthma and rhinitis comorbidity [Review – 38 refs]. *J Allergy Clin Immunol* 2000; **106**(5, Suppl): S201–S205.

98. Boulay ME, Boulet LP. The relationships between atopy, rhinitis and asthma: pathophysiological considerations [Review – 35 refs]. *Curr Opin Allergy Clin Immunol* 2003; **3**(1): 51–55.

99. Fuhlbrigge AL, Adams RJ. The effect of treatment of allergic rhinitis on asthma morbidity, including emergency department visits [Review – 31 refs]. *Curr Opin Allergy Clin Immunol* 2003; **3**(1): 29–32.

100. Knox AJ. How prevalent is aspirin induced asthma? *Thorax* 2002; **57**: 565–566.

101. Szczeklik A, Nizankowska E. Clinical features and diagnosis of aspirin induced asthma. *Thorax* 2000; **55**(Suppl): S42–S44.

102. Schatz M, Harden K, Forsythe A *et al*. The course of asthma during pregnancy, postpartum and with successive pregnancies: a prospective analysis. *J Allergy Clin Immunol* 1998; **81**: 509–517.

103. Gibson PG, Coughlan J, Wilson AJ *et al*. Self-management education and regular practitioner review for adults with asthma. The Cochrane Database of Systematic Reviews. The Cochrane Library No. 2, 2002.

104. Price D, Ryan D, Pearce L *et al.* The AIR Study: asthma in real life. *Asthma J* 1999; **4**(2): 74–77.

105. Busse W, Corren J, Lanier BQ *et al*. Omalizumab, anti-IgE recombinant humanized monoclonal antibody, for the treatment of severe allergic asthma. *J Allergy Clin Immunol* 2001; **108**: 184–190.

106. Larsen BB, Nielsen LP, Engelslatter R, Steinijans VW, Dahl R. Effect of ciclesonide on allergen challenge in subjects with bronchial asthma. *Allergy* 2003; **58**(207): 212.

Appendix 1 – Drugs

Short-acting β₂-agonists

Drug	Format	Trade name	Preparation	Strengths	Doses used in asthma	Comments	Side-effects
Salbutamol	Oral	Generic	Tablet	2, 4 mg	2–4 mg 3–4 times/day; child 2–6 years 1–2 mg 3–4 times/day, 6–12 years 2 mg 3–4 times/day	Not recommended	Tremor, tachycardia, hyperkalaemia
			Oral solution	2 mg/5 ml	2–4 mg 3–4 times/day; child < 2 years 100 mcg/kg 4 times/day*, 2–6 years 1–2 mg 3–4 times/day, 6–12 years 2 mg 3–4 times/day		
		Ventmax SR	M/R capsule	4, 8 mg	8 mg 2 times/day; child 3–12 years 4 mg 2 times/day		
		Ventolin	Syrup	2 mg/5 ml	2–4 mg 3–4 times/day; child < 2 years 100 mcg/kg 4 times/day*, 2–6 years 1–2 mg 3–4 times/day, 6–12 years 2 mg 3–4 times/day		
		Volmax	Tablet	4, 8 mg	8 mg 2 times/day; child 3–12 years 4 mg 2 times/day		
	Inhaled	Generic	MDI	100 mcg	100–200 mcg 3–4 times/day; child 100 mcg 3–4 times/day		Tremor, tachycardia (especially with nebulized preparations)

*Unlicenced according to the BNF (www.bnf.org)

Short-acting β₂-agonists (continued)

Drug	Format	Trade name	Preparation	Strengths	Doses used in asthma	Comments	Side-effects
Salbutamol	Inhaled	Generic	DPI	200, 400 mcg	200–400 mcg 3–4 times/day; child 200 mcg 3–4 times/day		
			Nebulizer solution	1, 2 mg/ml	2.5–5 mg 3–4 times/day; child < 18 months 1.25–2.5 mg 3–4 times/day*		
		Aerolin Autohaler	BAMDI	100 mcg	100–200 mcg 3–4 times/day; child 100 mcg 3–4 times/day		
		Airomir Inhaler	MDI	100 mcg	100–200 mcg 3–4 times/day; child 100 mcg 3–4 times/day		
		Airomir Autohaler	BAMDI	100 mcg	100–200 mcg 3–4 times/day; child 100 mcg 3–4 times/day		
		Asmasal Clickhaler	DPI	95 mcg	95–190 mcg 3–4 times/day; child 95 mcg 3–4 times/day		
		Salamol Easi-breathe Inhaler	BAMDI	100 mcg	100–200 mcg 3–4 times/day; child 100 mcg 3–4 times/day		
		Ventodisks	DPI	200, 400 mcg	200–400 mcg 3–4 times/day; child 200 mcg 3–4 times/day		
		Ventolin Evohaler	MDI	100 mcg	100–200 mcg 3–4 times/day; child 100 mcg 3–4 times/day		
		Ventolin Accuhaler	DPI	200 mcg	200 mcg 3–4 times/day		

*Unlicenced according to the BNF (www.bnf.org)

Short-acting β₂-agonists (continued)

Drug	Format	Trade name	Preparation	Strengths	Doses used in asthma	Comments	Side-effects
Salbutamol	Inhaled	Ventolin Nebules	Nebulizer solution	1, 2 mg/ml	2.5–5 mg 3–4 times/day	Dilute with sterile sodium chloride 0.9%	Tremor, tachycardia, hyperkalaemia
		Ventolin Respirator solution	Nebulizer solution	5 mg/ml	2.5–5 mg 3–4 times/day		
Terbutaline	Oral	Bricanyl	Tablet	5 mg	2.5–5 mg 3 times/day; child 7–15 years 2.5 mg 2–3 times/day	Not recommended	
			Syrup	1.5 mg/5 ml	2.5–5 mg 3 times/day; child < 7 years 75 mcg/kg 3 times/day, 7–15 years 2.5 mg 2–3 times/day		
		Bricanyl SA	M/R tablet	7.5 mg	7.5 mg 2 times/day		
		Monovent	Syrup	1.5 mg/5 ml	2.5–5 mg 3 times/day; child < 7 years 75 mcg/kg 3 times/day, 7–15 years 2.5 mg 2–3 times/day		
	Inhaled	Generic	Nebulizer solution	2.5 mg/ml	5–10 mg 2–4 times/day; child < 3 years 2 mg 2–4 times/day. 3–6 years 3 mg 2–4 times/day. 6–8 years 4 mg 2–4 times/day. > 8 years 5 mg 2–4 times/day		Tremor, tachycardia (especially with nebulized preparations)
		Bricanyl Inhaler	MDI	250 mcg	250–500 mcg 3–4 times/day		

Short-acting β₂-agonists (continued)

Drug	Format	Trade name	Preparation	Strengths	Doses used in asthma	Comments	Side-effects
Terbutaline	Inhaled	Bricanyl Turbohaler	DPI	500 mcg	250–500 mcg 3–4 times/day		
		Bricanyl Respules	Nebulizer solution	2.5 mg/ml	5–10 mg 2–4 times/day; child < 3 years 2 mg 2–4 times/day. 3–6 years 3 mg 2–4 times/day. 6–8 years 4 mg 2–4 times/day. > 8 years 5 mg 2–4 times/day		
		Bricanyl Respirator solution	Nebulizer solution	10 mg/ml	5–10 mg 2–4 times/day; child < 3 years 2 mg 2–4 times/day. 3–6 years 3 mg 2–4 times/day. 6–8 years 4 mg 2–4 times/day. > 8 years 5 mg 2–4 times/day	Dilute with sterile sodium chloride 0.9%	Tremor, tachycardia, hyperkalaemia
Bambuterol	Oral	Bambec	Tablet	10, 20 mg	10–20 mg nocte; not recommended for children	Not recommended	
Fenoterol + ipratropium	Inhaled	Duovent Inhaler	MDI	100 + 400 mcg	1–2 puffs 3–4 times/day; child > 6 years 1 puff 3 times/day	Combination products are only recommended if compliance is a problem	Tremor, tachycardia (especially with nebulized preparations), dry mouth, urinary retention, constipation, blurred vision, risk of glaucoma with nebulized formulations
		Duovent Autohaler	DPI	100 + 40 mcg	1–2 puffs 3–4 times/day; child > 6 years 1 puff 3 times/day		
		Duovent Nebulizer solution	Nebulizer solution	1.25 mg + 500 mcg/4 ml	1 vial up to 4 times daily; not recommended for children < 14 years		

Long-acting β₂-agonists

Drug	Format	Trade name	Preparation	Strengths	Doses used in asthma	Comments	Side-effects
Formoterol	Inhaled	Foradil	DPI	12 mcg	12–24 mcg 2 times/day; not recommended for children < 5 years	Not for relief of acute asthma attacks	Tremor, tachycardia, hyperkalaemia
		Oxis	DPI	6, 12 mcg	6–24 mcg 1–2 times/day (max 36 mg 2 times/day); child > 6 years 12 mcg 1–2 times/day		
Salmeterol	Inhaled	Serevent Inhaler	MDI	25 mcg	50–100 mcg 2 times/day; child > 4 years 50 mcg 2 times/day	Not for relief of acute asthma attacks	Tremor, tachycardia, paradoxical bronchospasm, hyperkalaemia
		Serevent Accuhaler	DPI	50 mcg	50–100 mcg 2 times/day; child > 4 years 50 mcg 2 times/day		
		Serevent Diskhaler	DPI	50 mcg	50–100 mcg 2 times/day; child > 4 years 50 mcg 2 times/day		

Anticholinergic bronchodilators

Drug	Format	Trade name	Preparation	Strengths	Doses used in asthma	Comments	Side-effects
Ipratropium	Inhaled	Generic	Nebulizer solution	250 mcg/ml	100–500 mcg up to 4 times/day; child 1 month–3 years 62.5–250 mcg up to 3 times/day* 3–14 years 100–500 mcg up to 3 times/day	Used to manage chronic asthma in patients who require high doses of corticosteroids	Dry mouth, urinary retention, constipation, blurred vision, risk of glaucoma with nebulized formulations (especially when given with salbutamol)
		Atrovent Inhaler	MDI	20, 40 mcg	20–80 mcg 3–4 times/day; child < 6 years 20 mcg 3 times/day, 6–12 years 20–40 mcg 3 times/day		
		Atrovent Aerocaps	DPI	40 mcg	40–80 mcg 3 times/day; not recommended for children < 12 years		
		Atrovent Autohaler	MDI	20 mcg	20–80 mcg 3–4 times/day; child < 6 years 20 mcg 3 times/day, 6–12 years 20–40 mcg 3 times/day		
		Atrovent Nebulizer solution	Nebulizer solution	250 mcg/ml	100–500 mcg up to 4 times/day; child 1 month–3 years 62.5–250 mcg up to 3 times/day* 3–14 years 100–500 mcg up to 3 times/day		
		Respontin	Nebulizer solution	250 mcg/ml	100–500 mcg up to 4 times/day; child 1 month–3 years 62.5–250 mcg up to 3 times/day* 3–14 years 100–500 mcg up to 3 times/day		*Unlicenced according to the BNF (www.bnf.org)

Anticholinergic bronchodilators (continued)

Drug	Format	Trade name	Preparation	Strengths	Doses used in asthma	Comments	Side-effects
Oxitropium	Inhaled	Oxivent Inhaler	MDI	100 mcg	200 mcg 2–3 times/day; not recommended for children	Used to manage chronic asthma in patients who require high doses of corticosteroids	Dry mouth, urinary retention, constipation, blurred vision
		Oxivent Autohaler	DPI	100 mcg	200 mcg 2–3 times/day; not recommended for children		
Tiotropium	Inhaled	Spiriva	DPI	18 mcg	18 mcg daily; not recommended for children and adolescents under 18 years old	Used for COPD. Consider in patients with combined asthma and COPD	Dry mouth, urinary retention, constipation, blurred vision, risk of glaucoma, pharyngitis, sinusitis, candidiasis, tachycardia (rare), difficulty in micturition (urinary retention in elderly men with prostatic carcinoma)

Methylxanthines

Drug	Format	Trade name	Preparation	Strengths	Doses used in asthma	Comments	Side-effects
Theophylline	Oral	Nuelin	Tablet	125 mg	125–250 mg 3–4 times/day; child 7–12 years 62.5–125 mg 3–4 times/day	Formulations are not interchangeable; take after food and swallow whole	**Plasma concentrations must be monitored;** multiple interactions with other drugs; nausea, tachycardia, hypokalaemia
			Liquid	60 mg/5 ml	120–240 mg 3–4 times/day; child 2–6 years 60–90 mg 3–4 times/day; 7–12 years 90–120 mg 3–4 times/day		
		Nuelin SA	M/R tablet	175, 250 mg	175–500 mg 2 times/day; child > 6 years 125–250 mg 2 times/day		
		Slo-Phyllin	M/R capsule	60, 125, 250 mg	250–500 mg 2 times/day; child 2–6 years 60–120 mg 2 times/day; 7–12 years 125–250 mg		
		Uniphyllin Continus	M/R tablet	200, 300, 400 mg	200–400 mg 2 times/day; child > 7 years 9 mg/kg 2 times/day (max 10–16 mg/kg 2 times/day)		
Aminophylline	Oral	Generic	Tablet	100 mg	100–300 mg 3–4 times/day	Formulations are not interchangeable; take after food and swallow whole	**Plasma concentrations must be monitored;** multiple interactions with other drugs; nausea, tachycardia, hypokalaemia
		Phyllocontin Continus	M/R tablet	100, 225, 350 mg	225–450 mg 2 times/day; smokers 350–700 mg 2 times/day; child > 3 years 6–12 mg/kg 2 times/day (max 13–20 mg/kg 2 times/day)		

Corticosteroids

Drug	Format	Trade name	Preparation	Strengths	Doses used in asthma	Comments	Side-effects
Beclometasone	Inhaled	Generic	MDI	50, 100, 200, 250 mcg	200 mcg 2 times/day or 100 mcg 3–4 times/day (initially 600–800 mcg/day in patients with severe asthma; max 500 mcg 4 times/day); child 50–100 mcg 2–4 times/day	Used to manage chronic asthma not controlled by short-acting β_2 stimulants	Oropharyngeal candidiasis, paradoxical bronchospasm, easy bruising, osteoporosis, cataracts (side-effects are dose and duration dependent)
			DPI	100, 200, 400 mcg	400 mcg 2 times/day or 200 mcg 3–4 times/day (max 800 mcg 2 times/day); child 100 mcg 2–4 times/day or 200 mcg 2 times/day		
		AeroBec Autohaler	BAMDI	50, 100, 250 mg	200 mcg 2 times/day or 100 mcg 3–4 times/day (initially 600–800 mcg/day in patients with severe asthma; max 500 mcg 4 times/day); child 50–100 mcg 2–4 times/day		
		Asmabec Clickhaler	DPI	50, 100, 250 mcg	200–400 mcg in 2–4 divided doses (initially 0.8–1.6 mg in 2–4 divided doses in patients with severe asthma; max 500 mcg 4 times/day); child 50–100 mcg 2–4 times/day		

Corticosteroids (continued)

Drug	Format	Trade name	Preparation	Strengths	Doses used in asthma	Comments	Side-effects
Beclometasone	Inhaled	Beclazone Easi-breathe Inhaler	BAMDI	50, 100, 250 mcg	200 mcg 2 times/day or 100 mcg 3–4 times/day (initially 600–800 mcg/day in patients with severe asthma; max 500 mcg 4 times/day): child 50–100 mcg 2–4 times/day		
		Becodisks	DPI	100, 200, 400 mcg	400 mcg 2 times/day or 200 mcg 3–4 times/day (max 800 mcg 2 times/day): child 100 mcg 2–4 times/day or 200 mcg 2 times/day		
		Becotide and Becloforte Inhalers	MDI	50, 100, 200, 250 mcg	200 mcg 2 times/day or 100 mcg 3–4 times/day (initially 600–800 mcg/day in patients with severe asthma; max 500 mcg 4 times/day): child 50–100 mcg 2–4 times/day		
		Qvar Inhaler	MDI	50, 100 mcg	50–200 mcg 2 times/day (max 400 mcg 2 times/day); not recommended for children	Lower doses of beclomethasone are given because of the propellant used in these formulations	
		Qvar Autohaler	BAMDI	50, 100 mcg	50–200 mcg 2 times/day (max 400 mcg 2 times/day); not recommended for children		

Corticosteroids (continued)

Drug	Format	Trade name	Preparation	Strengths	Doses used in asthma	Comments	Side-effects
Budesonide	Inhaled	Generic	DPI	200, 400 mcg	200–400 mcg every evening (max 800 mcg 2 times/day in severe asthma); child < 12 years 100–200 mcg 2 times/day (max 400 mcg 2 times/day in severe asthma) or 200–400 mcg every evening	Used to manage chronic asthma not controlled by short-acting β_2 stimulants	Oropharyngeal candidiasis, paradoxical bronchospasm, easy bruising, osteoporosis, cataracts (side-effects are dose and duration dependent)
		Pulmicort Inhaler	MDI	50, 200 mcg	200–400 mcg 2 times/day (max 1.6 mg/day in severe asthma); child 50–400 mcg 2 times/day (max 800 mcg/day in severe asthma)		
		Pulmicort Turbohaler	DPI	100, 200, 400 mcg	200–400 mcg every evening (max 800 mcg 2 times/day in severe asthma); child < 12 years 100–200 mcg 2 times/day (max 400 mcg 2 times/day in severe asthma) or 200–400 mcg every evening		
		Pulmicort Respules	Nebulizer suspension	250 mcg/ml	0.5–1 mg 2 times/day (1–2 mg 2 times/day in severe asthma); child 3 months to 12 years 250–500 mcg 2 times/day (0.5–1 mg 2 times/day in severe asthma)		

Corticosteroids (continued)

Drug	Format	Trade name	Preparation	Strengths	Doses used in asthma	Comments	Side-effects
Budesonide + formoterol	Inhaled	Symbicort Turbohaler	DPI	80 + 4.5 mcg; 160 + 4.5 mcg	1–2 puffs 1–2 times/day; not recommended for children and adolescents < 17 years	Used to manage chronic asthma not controlled by short-acting β_2 stimulants	Oropharyngeal candidiasis, paradoxical bronchospasm, easy bruising, osteoporosis, cataracts (side-effects are dose and duration dependent), tremor, tachycardia, hypokalaemia
Fluticasone	Inhaled	Flixotide Evohaler	MDI	25, 50, 125, 250 mcg	100–250 mcg 2 times/day (max 1 mg 2 times/day); child 4–16 years 50–100 mcg 2 times/day (max 200 mcg 2 times/day)	Used to manage Used to manage chronic asthma not controlled by short-acting β_2 stimulants	Oropharyngeal candidiasis, paradoxical bronchospasm, easy bruising, osteoporosis, cataracts (side-effects are dose and duration dependent)
		Flixotide Accuhaler	DPI	50, 100, 250, 500 mcg	100–250 mcg 2 times/day (max 1 mg 2 times/day); child 4–16 years 50–100 mcg 2 times/day (max 200 mcg 2 times/day)		
		Flixotide Diskhaler	DPI	50, 100, 250, 500 mcg	100–250 mcg 2 times/day (max 1 mg 2 times/day); child 4–16 years 50–100 mcg 2 times/day (max 200 mcg 2 times/day)		
		Flixotide Nebules	Nebulizer suspension	250 mcg/ml	0.5–2 mg 2 times/day; not recommended for children		

Corticosteroids (continued)

Drug	Format	Trade name	Preparation	Strengths	Doses used in asthma	Comments	Side-effects
Fluticasone + salmeterol	Inhaled	Seretide Evohaler	MDI	50 + 25 mcg; 125 + 25 mcg; 250 + 25 mcg	100 + 50 mcg to 500 + 50 mcg 2 times/day, reducing dose to once daily if control of asthma is maintained; not recommended for children < 12 years old	Used to manage chronic asthma not controlled by short-acting β_2 stimulants; combination products are only recommended if compliance is a problem	Oropharyngeal candidiasis, paradoxical bronchospasm, easy bruising, osteoporosis, cataracts (side-effects are dose and duration dependent), tremor, tachycardia, hyperkalaemia
		Seretide Accuhaler	DPI	100 + 50 mcg; 250 + 50 mcg; 500 + 50 mcg	100 + 50 mcg to 500 + 50 mcg 2 times/day reducing dose to once daily if control of asthma is maintained; not recommended for children < 12 years old		
Mometasone	Inhaled	Asmanex	MDI	200 + 400 mcg	200–400 mcg nocte increasing to 400 mcg twice daily if necessary; not recommended for children < 12 years old	Used to manage chronic asthma not controlled by short-acting β_2 stimulants	Oropharyngeal candidiasis, paradoxical bronchospasm, easy bruising, osteoporosis, cataracts (side-effects are dose and duration dependent)

Corticosteroids (continued)

Drug	Format	Trade name	Preparation	Strengths	Doses used in asthma	Comments	Side-effects
Prednisolone	Oral	Generic	Tablet	1, 5 mg	30–60 mg/day taken in the morning after breakfast for a few days to control acute asthma attacks; reduce dose gradually if asthma control is poor	Use high-dose inhaled corticosteroids when possible as they have fewer side-effects	Gastrointestinal (dyspepsia, ulceration), musculoskeletal (osteoporosis), endocrine (adrenal suppression, cushingoid effects likely with prolonged dosing > 7.5 mg/day, weight gain), neuropsychiatric (euphoria, depression), ophthalmic (glaucoma, cataracts)
			E/C tablet	2.5, 5 mg			
			Soluble tablet	5 mg			
		Deltacortril	E/C tablet	2.5, 5 mg			
		Precortisyl Forte	Tablet	25 mg			

Cromoglicate and related therapy

Drug	Format	Trade name	Preparation	Strengths	Doses used in asthma	Comments	Side-effects
Sodium cromoglicate	Inhaled	Generic	MDI	5 mg	10 mg 4 times/day (max 10 mg 6–8 times/day)	Regular use can reduce the incidence of asthma attacks and allow dosage reduction of bronchodilators and oral corticosteroids	Coughing, transient bronchospasm and throat irritation
			Nebulizer solution	10 mg/ml	20 mg 4 times/day (max 20 mg 6 times/day)		
		Cromogen Easi-breathe Inhaler	MDI	5 mg	10 mg 4 times/day (max 10 mg 6–8 times/day)		
		Intal Inhaler	MDI	5 mg	10 mg 4 times/day (max 10 mg 6–8 times/day)		
		Intal Spincaps	DPI	20 mg	20 mg 4 times/day (max 8 times/day)		
		Intal Nebulizer solution	Nebulizer solution	10 mg/ml	20 mg 4 times/day (max 20 mg 6 times/day)		
Sodium cromoglicate + salbutamol	Inhaled	Aerocrom Inhaler	MDI	1 mg + 100 mcg	2 puffs 4 times/day, not recommended for children	Not recommended	Coughing, transient bronchospasm and throat irritation, tremor, tachycardia, hyperkalaemia
Nedocromil sodium	Inhaled	Tilade Inhaler	MDI	2 mg	4 mg 4 times/day, not recommended for children > 6 years	Regular use can reduce the incidence of asthma attacks and allow dosage reduction of bronchodilators and oral corticosteroids	Coughing, transient bronchospasm and throat irritation

Ketotifen

Drug	Format	Trade name	Preparation	Strengths	Doses used in asthma	Comments	Side-effects
Ketotifen	Oral	Zaditen	Capsule	1 mg	1–2 mg 2 times/day: child > 2 years 1 mg 2 times/day	Continue with previous asthma treatment for at least 2 weeks after initiating ketotifen	Drowsiness, dry mouth, dizziness, CNS stimulation, weight gain
			Tablet	1 mg	1–2 mg 2 times/day: child > 2 years 1 mg 2 times/day		
			Elixir	1 mg/5 ml	1–2 mg 2 times/day: child > 2 years 1 mg 2 times/day		

Leukotriene receptor antagonists

Drug	Format	Trade name	Preparation	Strengths	Doses used in asthma	Comments	Side-effects
Montelukast	Oral	Singulair	Chewable tablet	4, 5 mg	10 mg nocte: child 2–5 years 4 mg nocte, 6–14 years 5 mg nocte	Not effective in relieving acute asthma attacks but used in prophylaxis of asthma	Gastrointestinal disturbances, dry mouth, thirst, hypersensitivity reactions, sleep disorders, Churg Strauss syndrome
			Tablet	10 mg	10 mg nocte: child 2–5 years 4 mg nocte, 6–14 years 5 mg nocte		
Zafirlukast	Oral	Accolate	Tablet	20 mg	20 mg 2 times daily; not recommended for children < 12 years	Not effective in relieving acute asthma attacks but used in prophylaxis of asthma	Gastrointestinal disturbances, headache, Churg Strauss syndrome

Appendix 2 – Useful Addresses and Websites

For health professionals

American Thoracic Society: www.thoracic.org

Association of Respiratory Nurse Specialists (ARNS):
www.arns.co.uk

British Society for Allergy and Clinical Immunology (BSACI):
www.bsaci.org

British Thoracic Society: www.brit-thoracic.org.uk

Canadian Thoracic Society: www.lung.ca/cts

European Respiratory Society: www.ersnet.org

General Practice Airways Group: www.gpiag.org

GINA: www.ginasthma.com

Hellenic Thoracic Society: www.hts.org.gr/ekdoseis_e.htm

Hong Kong Thoracic Society:
www.fmshk.com.hk/hkts/home.htm

IPCRG: www.theipcrg.org (for links to General Practice
Respiratory Groups in over 17 countries)

Medicines Partnership: www.medicines-partnership.org

National Heart, Lung, and Blood Institute: www.nhlbi.nih.gov

Oasys (Occupational Asthma):
www.occupationalasthma.com/

Scottish Thoracic Society:
www.rcpe.ac.uk/esd/clinical_standards/sts/sts_index.html

South African Thoracic Society: www.pulmonology.co.za

The Thoracic Society of Australia and New Zealand:
www.thoracic.org.au

World Health Organization: www.who.int/en/

For patients

European Federation of Allergy and Airways Diseases Patients'
Associations
EFA Central Office
Avenue Louise 327
1050 Brussels, Belgium
Tel.: +32 (0)2 646 9945
Fax: +32 (0)2 646 4116
E-mail: efaoffice@skynet.be
www.efanet.org

Austria: lungenunion@chello.at
Belgium: astmafonds.gent@skynet.be
astmastichting@belgacom.net
www.fares.be
Bulgaria: simona_ralcheva@abv.bg
Czech Republic: cipa@volny.cz
www.cipa.cz
Denmark: jg@astma-allergi.dk
www.astma-allergi.dk
Finland: international@allergia.com
www.allergia.com
France: bbbj@club-internet.fr / bruneliane@aol.com
www.ffaair.org
Germany: info@daab.de
www.daab.de
Greece: receiver@allergyped.gr
www.allergyped.gr
Hungary: strj@helka.iif.hu
www.resphun.com
Ireland: asthma@indigo.ie
www.asthmasociety.ie

Italy: federasma@fsm.it
    www.federasma.org
Lithuania: jolantakudzyte@omni.lt
Norway: post@lhl.no
    www.lhl.no
Portugal: www.ciberconceito.com/apa/
    apa@ciberconceito.com
Serbia and Montenegro: vesnapetr@ptt.yu
    www.yudah.org.yu
Slovenia: dpbs@siol.net
    www.astma-info.com
Spain: maeve@mundo-r.com
    www.accessible.org/asga
Sweden: info@astmaoallergiforbundet.se
    www.astmaoallergiforbundet.se
Switzerland: info@ahaswiss.ch
    www.ahaswiss.ch
The Netherlands: b.talens@betuwe.net
    info@astmafonds.nl
    www.astmafonds.nl
United Kingdom: National Asthma Campaign
    mdockrell@asthma.org.uk
    www.asthma.org.uk

British Lung Foundation (BLF)
enquiries@blf-uk.org
www.lunguk.org

Training organizations

National Respiratory Training Centre: www.nrtc.org.uk
Respiratory Education Centre: www.respiratoryetc.com

Index

Note: Abbreviations used in this index can be found on page (vii)

As Asthma is the subject of this book, all index entries refer to Asthma unless otherwise indicated. Page numbers followed by 'f' indicate figures; page numbers followed by 't' indicate tables. This index is in letter-by-letter order, whereby spaces and hyphens in main entries are excluded from the alphabetization process.

Rapid Reference

A major new series of pocketbooks

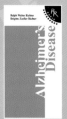

Ralph Walter Richter
Brigitte Zoeller Richter
Alzheimer's Disease

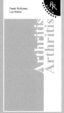

Frank McKenna
Lee Simon
Arthritis

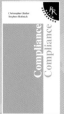

Christopher Butler
Stephen Rollnick
Compliance

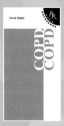

David Halpin
COPD

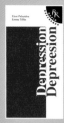

Eleni Palazidou
Lenna Tillim
Depression

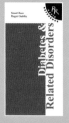

Stuart Ross
Roger Gadsby
Diabetes & Related Disorders

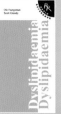

Olu Famgetman
Scott Grundy
Dyslipidaemia

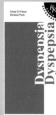

Emad El-Omar
Richard Peek
Dyspepsia

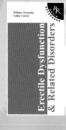

William Alexander
Culley Carson
Erectile Dysfunction & Related Disorders

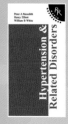

Peter A Meredith
Henry Elliott
William B White
Hypertension & Related Disorders

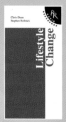

Chris Dean
Stephen Rollnick
Lifestyle Change

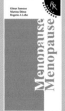

Gösta Samsioe
Martins Dören
Rogerio A Lobo
Menopause

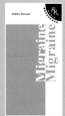

Andrew Dowson
Migraine

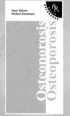

Stuart Ralston
Michael Kleerekoper
Osteoporosis

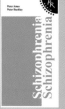

Peter Jones
Peter Buckley
Schizophrenia

Mosby

www.elsevierhealth.com

ELSEVIER SCIENCE